Simply
Nourished

By Amanda Harvey

www.THE NOBLE NUTRITIONIST.com

Published By
The Noble Nutritionist LTD
Narre Warren North, Victoria Australia 3804

First Publication in 2014
Copyright © Amanda J Harvey

ebook ISBN 978-163315807-8
Paperback ISBN 978-1500114367

Cover by Heli Herrera
Cover photo by Ken Pryer http://www.kenpryor.com/

Life is not complex.
We are complex.
Life is simple, and the simple thing is
the right thing

Oscar Wilde

ACKNOWLEDGMENTS

The first person I would like to acknowledge is my husband, Jesse. You are an astounding man and it is with your support that this book exists. Thank you for dedicating hours of your time, reading, editing and re-reading, until this book was complete. Thank you for your encouragement, you helped me believe in myself and reminded me that anything is possible, all you have to do is create it. I adore you, not only as my husband, but also as my best friend. I love you and I cannot picture my life without you in it.

My loving parents. Mum- your talent in the kitchen has been an inspiration to me. I feel lucky to have grown up with a Mother who has a passion for cooking like you. Every meal you put together was, and still is, made with love. Not only was it delicious, it was also nutritious. I learnt my cooking skills from you, so thank you for teaching me my way around the kitchen. You have such a kind heart and all that I can ask is that I am as caring as a Mother as you were to us. You always put our needs first and generosity like yours is something I aspire to.

Dad- I don't know anyone who is as hard working as you are. Your are committed and demand perfection with any task that you take on.

I wouldn't be where I am today if I hadn't acquired this asset from you. When I see you with your grandson, it reminds me of the love that you gave to my brothers and I as we were growing up. Thank you for your affection, I feel loved by you and know that you will always be there for me, no matter what.

My two parents are pretty amazing. Even through the tough times, together you showed strength and made everyday bright and sunny. I love you both so much, thank you for all that you have done for me, and continue to do.

I would like to acknowledge someone who open handedly volunteered his time. Stephen, you were so kind to offer your assistance. I appreciate the effort and time you put into my very first book, I couldn't have done it without your editing skills so thank you for being so kind.

Last but not least, I would like to acknowledge the farmers. The ones who farm ethically and organically, the way all food should be produced. This allows us to build health and vitality and I am forever grateful for that. Food that is grown naturally, allows for optimum flavour so thank you for making food wonderful.

FORWARD

I am a food enthusiast. I spend a lot of my time in the kitchen and love planning meals and creating new recipes. I also enjoy dining out and trying new restaurants. I live in Melbourne, Australia and am lucky to have fantastic cafes and restaurants nearby. At the end of the week my husband and I have shared many outings together, catching up on the activities in each others lives whilst enjoying delicious food. We tend to stick to places who source their food locally and serve organic, seasonal produce that has been raised ethically. Food that is in a natural state, it has not been sprayed with chemicals, genetically modified or fed an unnatural diet. This is, what I call 'real' food.

For me, it is important to know where my food comes from. I want to know how the crops are grown and I care deeply about the treatment of animals. I do not tolerate factory farming and to be honest, due to the treatment of some animals, I could easily become vegan. However, the nutrients that animals provide is vital to a thriving human body, so instead I choose to be particular of where I buy my produce. I shop at farmers markets, that way I can deal directly with the farmer. We have a good chat about how they manage their farms, what they use to keep pests away and how they house their animals. I know that the produce has not been treated with harmful pesticides, chemicals or antibiotics and that the animals have a good quality of life. Things that I cannot find at the farmers markets, I buy organic from the local health food store. The only item I buy from the supermarket is toilet paper, which I buy in bulk. With less money going into supermarkets and non-organic growers I am able to better support what I believe in, organic local growers. As support grows, so will the demand and products will become more widely available for the general public.

I practice yoga and love the great outdoors, I do not own a house and have not lived in one place for longer than a year, I shop at the local op-shops and try to buy recycled goods as much as possible. I avoid chemicals by steering clear of cosmetics and use aromatherapy and natural products, like coconut oil instead. I am a conscious omnivore and I eat local, organic, preferably biodynamic, real food. I have a Diploma in Nutrition, and my passion is to share with others how to adopt a traditional diet. I am lucky to be married to the most wonderful man I have ever set eyes on, he is my best friend, my soul mate and together we have a beautiful son Jasper, born June of 2013.

Dedicated to Jesse and Jasper,
you always make me smile

Simply Nourished
Contents

INTRODUCTION

Gone are the days where all food provides nourishment. We are so overwhelmed with misinformation and crazy fads that feeding ourselves has become impossible. In this book we will venture on a journey of discovering what real food is. If you wish, this knowledge can define a lifestyle change for you. With this information you will have the tools to build the healthy body you desire. These tools will be with you for a lifetime and most of all, it is an enjoyable journey, a journey into a world of delicious, real food!

The body thrives on traditional foods. These are foods that are in their most natural state possible. The same foods that we were eating millennia ago. Foods such as full fat dairy, pastured animal produce, bone broths, properly prepared nuts and ancient grains, fruit and vegetables that are in season and fermented foods and beverages. I believe that there is no particular diet that we should abide by. We are all different and our bodies respond to food differently from one another, finding what works for you is your main priority.

We all have developed habits around food. Some habits are healthy, and these are the ones to hold on to. On the other hand, some can be detrimental to your health and need to be changed. In this book you will get the chance to evaluate your habits, and learn to recognise both the good and the bad. You will learn about the effects that your choices have on your body, and how they impact your life. I will guide you to make small changes in your lifestyle that will enable you to build a healthy body and reach your desired goals. These changes and results will last a lifetime.

BUILDING DIRECTION

Direction: The course that must be taken in order to reach a destination
Goals: The object of a person's ambition or effort; an aim or desired result

To accomplish a goal you must first know which path to take and to do this, you need direction. It is up to you to determine what your health goals are. There are no limits when choosing your goals, they can be anything from losing weight, breaking a sugar habit or learning how to cook nutritious meals. Whatever you wish for yourself and your life you can have it. So right now, stop reading, get a piece of paper and pen and write down your goals, do not just think about them, or make a mental note, make an actual note! Writing down your goals is one of the best ways to make them become reality in your life. Once you have written down your goals, put the paper somewhere that you will read it at least twice a day. I have mine stuck on my bedside table, that way when I wake up in the morning, I read what I have set out for myself to achieve. I find this works well as it is a great reminder of what I want in my life. Another way is to set an alarm on your phone or computer. With the alarm add a note that lists your goals, do this at some point in the morning so you can begin your day with your goals in mind.

3

Over the next seven days I recommend that you create a food journal. Your food journal will allow you to evaluate your total food consumption by recording everything you eat and drink. As you continue through the book you will become aware of the impact that different types of food have on your body. You can take a look at your existing food intake and can make adjustments where you see fit. Remember to also include beverages. It is best to have the journal with you at all times though, so that you do not miss out on recording anything. Your phone or a notepad could be a better option for you. It is important to include absolutely everything that you eat each day, even if it is a tiny bite of a piece of cake. It is really important to look at the foods you are eating so that you can make adjustments for your new lifestyle change. Continue to eat the foods that you would normally eat for now, otherwise it will be very difficult to make the lifestyle change.

In your food journal also note the time of day that you consumed each meal or snack and your feelings and emotions before, during and after eating. This will allow you to recognise the reasons you eat. Are you eating because you are hungry and need energy? Is it out of comfort because you are feeling down? Or perhaps you saw an advertisement on television that made you want to eat that particular food? Whatever the reason, understanding why you eat is an important aspect to your lifestyle change.

4

We can get caught up on how much we weigh, or what size jeans we wear, and we are unaware of the negative impact that this has on us. The first step to being happy with your body is to accept it. There are things that you can change, like losing weight for instance, but there are also things that will remain the same, such as the structure of your bones, and thus, the shape of your body. We all come in many forms and sizes, that is what is so wonderful about the human body. Your body is unique to you, so give up comparing and embrace the beauty you have. Forget weighing yourself, weight fluctuates often, and for numerous reasons. Instead, focus on building a healthy body through this journey into a traditional food diet, once you begin it, the results you desire will sure follow.

If you are wishing to lose weight, the best way to do this is gradually. A gradual weight loss will not leave you feeling deprived and the results will last. When weight is lost too quickly, it is often due to a quick fix or fad diet. These weight loss tactics usually result in weight coming back, and often in larger amounts. In my book you will learn how to lose weight gradually and maintain your ideal weight forever by simply nourishing your body through eating traditional foods. This is going to be the factor that will help you reach your goals.

THIS IS NOT A DIET

I dislike the word 'diet' due to what it has come to represent in our modern western world. When we hear this word we immediately think, restriction, deprivation and limiting food in order to lose weight. In fact, the actual definition of the word diet is "food and drink regularly provided or consumed."[1] So when you see the word diet throughout the book, just remember that I am using this definition. You have likely heard of many quick fix programs, or so-called "diets" that require you to restrict your food consumption in some way or another, such as cutting out a particular food group, using meal replacement shakes and bars or consuming nothing but juices. These are fads meaning that they are 'short-lived.' They may show results initially, but the results rarely last and in many cases, extra weight gain can be the outcome. These fads have a detrimental impact on your body both physically and mentally. You are often left feeling tired, run-down, hungry, irritable, depressed and have trouble thinking straight. I want you to be aware of these 'fad diets'. They are not a lifestyle, but rather a quick fix to short term weight loss. It seems absurd to live in such an unpleasant way; and it is not worth the effort.

Unfortunately the amount of misinformation in the media makes it difficult to know what foods to eat and what foods to avoid. You are probably wondering:

"What kind of diet should I be consuming?" The answer is simple, one that includes real food. Real foods contain important macronutrients and micronutrients that the body needs in order to thrive. Throughout this book I will educate you about these food constituents. I will discuss what is needed for a healthy life and explain the foods that provide the best sources. You will also learn the foods that you should avoid. By the end of this book the choices you make around food will be simple. You will know how, what and why you eat the foods that you do and how to incorporate these foods into your diet.

The first step in your lifestyle change is to accept that it takes time for your body to adapt to your new diet. This will be a pleasant journey and one that you will want to continue on forever. You will feel amazing and most importantly, you have done this by nurturing your body and mind with real food.

CONTROVERSIAL CARBOHYDRATES

Carbohydrates supply the body with energy. There are many different types of carbohydrates and choosing the right ones is important.

Carbohydrates come in three forms[2];

Sugar
Sugar is the simplest forms of carbohydrate. It occurs naturally in some foods, including fruits, vegetables, and dairy products. Fructose is the main sugar found in fruit, sucrose (which is fructose and glucose together) is the sugar found in table sugar and milk sugar is lactose. Fructose in excess amounts has been shown to be very harmful to the body in many ways. (more on this later in the chapter.)

Starch
Starch is made of sugar units bonded together. It occurs naturally in vegetables, grains, and cooked dry beans and peas.

Fibre
Fibre also is made of sugar units bonded together but our digestive tract cannot break the bonds. Fruits, vegetables, grains are among foods that

8

are naturally rich in fibre. Fibre is necessary for gastrointestinal health and a very important part of the diet.

The amount of carbohydrates a person needs will depend on many things. Each person has different energy demands and thus their carbohydrate intake will vary. Someone who is very physically active will require more carbohydrates than someone who is not; for example, a tennis player requires more energy than a golfer and needs to adjust their diet accordingly.

There are two types of fuel sources the body will use. One is fat the other is carbohydrates which includes both sugar as well as starches such as white potatoes, white rice, cereal and bread- even most gluten free bread. If its available the body will choose to use sugar and starch as its primary energy source. It will not dive into its fat stores until all of the sugar and starch has been used. If the sugar does not get used up it will be stored as fat.

This is important to keep in mind, not only if you plan to lose weight (a low intake of carbohydrates will expedite weight loss), but it is the key to building an efficiently running body. Think of carbohydrates as the opening act and fats as the main event. I do not suggest that you start counting the grams of carbohydrates you eat, but it may help to familiarise yourself with the carbohydrate content in foods. Everyone's body has different energy needs, and you will need to pay close attention to yours and work out what it requires. It may take some experimenting, but soon enough you will ascertain how much carbohydrate your body needs. Keep in mind that with your activity level the amount of energy from food, in the form of carbohydrates, fats and protein, will change day to day. A more physically active day will require more energy from food than a day of sitting on the beach for example.

Grains, friend or foe?

There is much debate on whether grains should be a part of our diet. It has been shown that grains containing gluten (found in wheat, rye, spelt, bulgar and kamut) can cause problems in the body, and in some cases without you even knowing it.

I can understand if you are a little confused- for so long it has been recommended that sixty percent of your dietary calories consist of carbohydrates, and mostly in the form of whole grains. This amount is extremely high. I recommend that your intake be much lower. Grains are high in carbohydrates and low in fat and protein, simply put, they are nutrient poor. You want to fuel your body with nutrient rich foods, ones that are higher in fat and protein. Not only do these taste better, but the body runs more efficiently on them. They provide much greater satiety signals, keeping you fuller for longer, meaning you are more likely to lose or maintain weight. You will have more energy and generally feel better overall. Grains do provide you with vitamins and minerals such as vitamin B, iron, magnesium, folate and fibre. However, you can obtain these nutrients from other sources. A traditional diet containing meat, oil, dairy, nuts, seeds, fruit and vegetables will provide these nutrients in abundance.

By avoiding grains in the diet you can avoid the health issues related high dietary carbohydrate. In very basic terms carbohydrates of any form get digested in simple sugars, these simple sugars will stick to the proteins in your body. Too much sugar stuck to proteins makes them work improperly, they literally get sticky! If you have too many proteins with too much sugar stuck to them for a long time, it will make you sick.

David Perlmutter, a renowned neurologist, explains the detrimental effects that grains can have, especially on the brain. In his book 'Grain Brain', David provides scientific research indicating that grains destroy your brain and can contribute to the many diseases such as dementia, ADHD, epilepsy, anxiety, depression, decreased libido, headaches and much more. For further reading on this topic I highly recommend his book.

What Carbohydrates Should You Choose?

Over the last few thousand years our consumption of grains has increased due to our shift from nomadic lifestyle to an agricultural lifestyle. Highly processed, genetically modified grains have only been a part of our diet for the past sixty years or so since the advent of industrialised agriculture after WWII. The modern crossbred wheat grain that has been introduced into todays diet shows little resemblance to the wild einkorn variety that our Neolithic ancestors consumed seasonally, or our more recent ancestors grew in their small farms.

To avoid these genetically modified, high gluten grains you are better to choose gluten free ancient grains, such as amaranth, buckwheat, millet and quinoa. All vegetables are gluten free and provide a good source of complex carbohydrates. Vegetables such as sweet potato, yams, pumpkin, squash, turnips, carrots and parsnips are higher in carbohydrates than broccoli, cauliflower, beans, peas, asparagus, kale and lettuce. When baking, coconut and nut flours are fantastic options to replace wheat flours. These can be used to make bread and other baked goods.

How to Properly Prepare Grains

If you choose to include grains they must be prepared correctly.

Most grains contain a substance called phytic acid. This substance is what plants use to store phosphorus, a nutrient necessary for plant growth. It is present in almost all seeds. Phosphorus in this form is not bioavailable to humans because we lack the enzyme phytase that is required to separate phosphorus from the phytic acid. Phytic acid binds to other minerals as well, such as calcium, iron, zinc and magnesium. It also binds to B vitamins. Binding with phytic acid blocks absorption of these nutrients and can contribute to a mineral deficiency. For proper absorption of these important minerals and vitamins, phytic acid needs to be removed from the grains[3].

To remove phytic acid, the grains need to be properly prepared, fermenting or sprouting them will accomplish this.

Fermentation is done by allowing them to soak from a minimum of twelve hours, and up to twenty-four hours. Simply place them into a bowl, filling the bowl with water and adding a small amount (about 1 tbsp) of a lacto-fermented or acidic product such as yoghurt, buttermilk, raw milk, kefir, lemon juice, or apple cider vinegar. Let this sit on the counter for twelve to twenty-four hours. It really is an easy process and does not take much effort at all.

Another way to avoid phytic acid is by consuming sprouted grains, seeds and nuts. Sprouting allows the grain to germinate which means phytic acid will not be present. You can buy sprouted bread, flour, nuts and seeds at health food stores.

Do I Eat Grains?

I personally have a gluten sensitivity. When I eat it I get a headache, feel bloated and lethargic and my eczema breaks out, and takes up to four weeks to disappear. For this reason I avoid gluten containing grains. I prefer to eat food that is going to nourish my body so I consume a diet that is high in fat and protein and low in carbohydrates. Therefore, I eat minimal grains and legumes. I may have some brown rice or lentils here and there, but this happens infrequently. When I do consume grains and legumes, I make sure that they have been properly prepared, so that I am not leaching nutrients from my body. I avoid modern wheat and choose gluten free ancient grains instead. On special occasions, such as a birthday, I would make a cake with a sprouted gluten free flour or better yet, coconut and nut flours. Bread in my home is made fresh with blanched almond meal (blanching neutralises the phytic acid). I create many flavours from sweet potato to zucchini.

14

Topped with cheese, avocado, sauerkraut or seasonal vegetables, it is a meal that my family always looks forward to. If you feel that you may be sensitive to gluten and want to find out how you feel without it, an elimination diet can help. Simply eliminate gluten containing foods from your diet for sixty days. Once the sixty days are over, eat foods containing gluten and notice how you feel. This can be done with any type of food that you may be sensitive too, such as dairy or eggs. Discovering our sensitivities will decrease inflammation in the body which will have a huge impact on our overall health.

Another grain free option is buckwheat. This is often mistaken for wheat but it is actually related to the rhubarb family. Buckwheat has a rich nutty flavour and is both gluten and grain free. It comes as a flour, which can be substituted for wheat flour in muffins, cakes, pancakes, bread and cookies. It also comes as groats which resembles rice. This can be used in replacement of oats, bread crumbs or cereal. Buckwheat contains phytic acid so be sure that it has been properly prepared. You can purchase sprouted buckwheat, this means you do not have to soak the groats or flour, it comes ready to be used.

Simple Carbohydrates

Sugar is any simple carbohydrate such as glucose, fructose, galactose, dextrose, maltose or any pair of these simple sugars. For example, sucrose (table sugar) is composed of two simple sugars, glucose & fructose, while lactose (milk sugar) is made of glucose & galactose.[4]

Humans have evolved a digestive tract that did not have to deal with sugar regularly as it is rarely found in large quantities in the wild. Our ancestors may have found some honey, or an apple tree in season, and would have had a large sugar load once or twice a year, but otherwise sugar was not a regular part of the diet.

Our physiology has evolved to metabolise a small amount of sugar per day before it starts to play havoc on our system. Your sugar consumption can add up very quickly because it is present in many modern foods. For example, a chocolate bar, bowl of cereal, can of coke and glass of fruit juice, all have at least twenty-five grams of sugar each. This a large amount of sugar for just one serving and for the entire day for that matter. Also, foods containing high amounts of sugar generally do not contain a lot of fat and protein and therefore, are lower in nutrients.

Your fruit intake also contributes to your sugar consumption so keep this in mind when thinking about your daily intake of sugar. Because fruit contains vitamins and fibre, it is a better choice than processed sugary foods. Fibre slows the absorption of sugar which keeps insulin levels stable and helps prevent drops in energy. I do not think that fruit needs to be eliminated from your diet, but I do not see it as essential. If you are not a big fan of fruit, this is fine, as long as you eat a wide variety of vegetables and other nutrient rich foods. Personally I only eat fruit and vegetables that are in season. I find that imported out of season fruit and vegetables are very bland and lacking in flavour.

Do not be fooled by the word 'natural sweetener'. Even though the sweetener comes from a natural source, it still effects the body the same way as cane sugar. Natural sweeteners include types such as agave, honey, coconut nectar, molasses, rice malt or maple syrup; they all contain sugars.

When I bake treats I use honey or maple syrup. I like the flavour and find them extremely sweet so I only use tiny amounts. For special occasions I may use coconut sugar. I use brown rice syrup when I want to make something fructose free. Just remember that every little bit of sugar counts and the less you eat the less you will want. If you were to ask me what I consider to be the most important health tip my answer would be to cut down on sugar as it disrupts our whole being.

Basically, when it comes down to it, a sugar is a sugar. Yes there are better choices to make, for example, choosing organic raw honey instead of agave syrup, but honey still contains sugar. Even though it is natural and contains some nutrients, it is still metabolised by the body the same way as cane sugar. My recommendations of daily sugar consumption is no more than 6-7 teaspoons or 28.8-33.6 grams, the less the better, especially if you suffer with an autoimmune disease. This includes the sugar found in fruit. About 2-3 servings of fruit would contain this much but of course fruit is a much better choice over a sweetener of any sort. If your diet is made up of a lot of packaged foods (including condiments) the grams of sugar will add up extremely quickly, as they are often ladened with sugar. I personally eat around 5-15 grams of sugar most days. I find that my body thrives on this small amount and I feel at my best when I keep it low. I don't eat much fruit and when I do I make sure it is in season. In replacement of fruit I get my nutrients by eating plenty of vegetables, I like to do this and treat myself to a few squares of extra dark chocolate (85%-92%) instead.

A little on rice malt syrup

Rice malt syrup is made from fermented, cooked rice. It is very sweet, so just a tiny amount is needed. The reason for this is it contains only maltose and glucose, it is fructose free. The body is much better at metabolising glucose than fructose. Fructose is metabolised by the liver, any excess amounts get converted to fat very easily. In saying this, it is still important to keep any form of sweetener to a minimum.

How sugar is making us fat and sick

In ancient times sugar was not widely available so it was consumed infrequently. Nowadays it is easily accessible and is a contributor to most of the health problems seen in modern western society. It is hidden in most packaged and processed food and beverages, and if you do not eat whole foods, sugar is almost impossible to avoid. Sugar has been linked to heart disease, diabetes, cancer, a weakened immune system and contributes to difficulties in losing and maintaining weight which can lead to obesity.

From 1910-1970 saturated animal fats were decreased in the average western diet.[5] It is widely assumed that saturated fat is the cause of diseases such as heart disease, obesity and diabetes. However, although our intake of saturated fat has decreased, these diseases are still on the rise. What is the reason for this? Because saturated fat was considered unhealthy, a 'low-fat' diet was encouraged. When fat is removed from food, it lacks flavour and sugar is used to replace the fat to enhance the flavour and texture of food. As fat

19

decreased in the diet, sugar consumption increased proportionately. Emerging independent research indicates that sugar, along with seed oils, is the main contributor to the dietary diseases of western society.[6,7,8,9]

Not only does an excess consumption of sugar lead to heart disease, obesity and diabetes, it also has other harmful effects on the body;

- Depletes the body of B vitamins. These are important for many functions such as, energy metabolism, making red blood cells, carrying oxygen around the body, producing hormones and maintaining healthy skin and nerves[10]
- Suppresses the immune system making you more prone to sickness
- Causes inflammation which has been linked to cancer[11]
- Disrupts energy levels causing peaks and dips of energy throughout the day causing you to become irritable and thus interferes with your daily life and happiness
- Upsets the balance of calcium and phosphorus which can lead to bone loss and tooth decay[12]
- Upsets the balance of hormones that are responsible for producing satiety signals in the body, this leads to overeating because you never feel satisfied after meals [13]

If losing weight is a goal of yours, an excess consumption of sugar in your diet may be the reason you are not getting closer to reaching your goals. Sugar interferes with the function of the body's hormones that naturally act as a satiety switch. When we eat food with too much sugar, the bodies normal "fullness gage" is rendered nonfunctional. [14]

There are three main hormones that control satiety in our bodies, and they are activated by different nutrients. When we eat protein and fat, our stomach releases the hormone Cholecystokinin (CCK) which tells us that we are full and we stop eating. When we eat carbohydrates, our pancreas releases the hormone insulin which plays an important role in glucose metabolism and satiety. Leptin is another hormone that controls appetite, it is released by fat cells and effectively tells the brain how much fat we have saved up. Too much sugar derails all three of these satiety hormones so we feel hungry, and eat more. Consuming too much sugar, especially in the form of fructose (which is present not only in table sugar but also in natural sweeteners such as maple syrup and honey), bypasses the normal satiety signals. Fructose is metabolised by the liver and the liver is fantastic at converting fructose into fat. The fat circulates in the blood stream in the form of triglycerides and disrupts those important appetite-suppressing hormones preventing them from doing their job. This

21

means you do not know that you are full and in fact, you feel even hungrier which causes you to eat more, and usually more of the sweet stuff, as a result, you gain weight. The cycle continues and it becomes very difficult to lose or even maintain weight.[15]

How To Quit A Sugar Habit

Now that you are aware of the detrimental effects excess sugar has on your health, I am sure you are ready to reduce your consumption. Sugar has probably been a part of your diet for many years now, consuming it will be a habit, possibly an addiction. As with any change, it will take time for you to adjust to the reduction of sugar in your diet and this is completely normal. There are two ways I suggest that will help you to decrease your sugar consumption:

Option 1 - Cold Turkey
> You can eliminate sugar from your diet altogether for six weeks, and then slowly introduce it back, in a healthy amount. This means no sugar whatsoever, not even fruit.

Option 2 - Gradual Decrease and Replacements
> You can slowly decrease your sugar intake until your reach a healthy amount. This can be done by cutting down your sugar portions. For example, if you eat snacks containing sugar,

decrease the amount that you eat each day. Or you can make replacements, for example, swap a muesli bar (yes even these have sugar) for a piece of fruit and slice of cheese or replace milk chocolate with good quality 75%+ dark chocolate. When choosing chocolate, make sure you get one that does not contain soy lecithin (more on soy later in the book), choose one with cacao, cacao butter and a form of sweetener (or no sweetener if you prefer the extreme dark kind). 75% chocolate will have around twenty-five grams of sugar per 100 grams, the higher the cacao percentage, the less sugar. Due to the richness of the cacao, you will not eat a lot of it at a time, unlike the super sweet milk chocolate that has you coming back for more and more.

The option that you choose is entirely up to you. You know what would suit you best and perhaps you might give both a try. I personally find that the second option works best as the first one can leave you feeling a little deprived. Remember that you will be increasing your fat consumption and therefore, you will feel satisfied after meals, this will help to reduce your sugar cravings.

Choices Around Sugar

Here are a few ways that will make reducing sugar a little easier.

Prepare your mind for the change

Before you begin kicking your sugar habit you need to have the right mindset. Tell yourself that you are taking control of your health and that decreasing your sugar consumption is a major component of that. It may be tough at times, but in time, you will no longer 'need' sugar to feel satisfied.

Remove habits associated with eating sugar

Do you find that when you are at the movies or have found a comfy spot to read a favourite book, that sweet treat is already sitting beside you, ready to be devoured? Believe it or not, you can still enjoy the movie or book without consuming a sugar filled snack. This requires a break in your usual routine, and some getting used to. Once you have made the change, you will be just as happy without the sugar snacks as you were with them.

Years ago, before I realised how detrimental sugar was, my husband and I would habitually go to the movies and order a large popcorn and a bag of sugary snacks, I would consume a whole packet of chocolate crunchy chocettes, not just one or two pieces, the whole packet. By the end of the movie, my head would be thumping and I would be shaking from the sugar rush. What I found insane, is that even after all that chocolate I was still hungry, so we would eat more. Sugar really is a poison and it was times like these that made me realise that. Now, we make our own popcorn and take some good quality chocolate instead. I swapped the milk chocolate for darker varieties, starting with 60% and gradually moving towards 85%, I even enjoy the richness of 90% now. Part of our movie routine was the snacks associated with it, but making the change to healthy choices has only left us with a bit more cash, and no sugar crash at the end of the film, contributing to our healthier lifestyle.

It is really easy to modify your food choices so that your sugar intake stays in control. Be sure to read the label of any packaged foods to see exactly what it contains.

Remove sugar from your house and workplace

This is a great way of removing the temptation and will help you to break your sugar habit. If you do not have easy access to it, you will not be as tempted to eat it.

Here are a list of foods that are best avoided and
alternative ways to replace them;

Flavoured beverages (sodas and juices)-
The best choice of beverages are
water, kombucha, kefir, coconut milk,
unsweetened nut milks or full fat raw
milk from grass-fed cows. Avoid
flavoured water, soft drinks (even diet)
flavoured milk and fruit juices. You may
think that fruit juices are healthy because
they are made from fruit, however, the
amount of sugar in them is surprising.
You could max out your total daily
consumption from just one small bottle of
fruit juice. Even freshly squeezed juices
contain large amounts of sugar.

Replacements- squeeze a little
lemon into your water and drink full fat
milk. I have delicious chocolate
milkshake and hot chocolate recipes, that
really hit the spot. When consuming
fruit, make smoothies instead, these
contain the whole fruit and include the
fibre so you do not get the sugar rush and
you also get more nutrients. Remember
to keep your fruit intake to no more than

three servings per day. Make green juices using vegetables. Use dairy, nut and coconut milk or water to bulk up the smoothie. Introduce kombucha into your diet. This is a raw, fermented, probiotic, and naturally carbonated tea. You will find more information on kombucha, including instructions on how to brew your own batch in the comfort of your own home on my website. (www.thenoblenutritionsit.com)

Confectionery

Such as chocolate bars, biscuits, candy and ice-cream. These foods offer no nutritional value whatsoever and are full of sugar, rancid vegetable fats and additives.

Replacements- swap candy milk chocolate for real dark chocolate. Remember to choose one that is seventy-five percent cacao or more, otherwise the sugar can still be quite high. Swap conventional ice-cream for a full fat natural yoghurt, avoid ones with sugar or additives. You can also try making your own ice-cream, using less sweetener will make it a healthy option. My recipe for

'Honey and Macadamia Nut Ice Cream'
is also online.

Snack Bars

Almost always have a sugar of
some sort added. There are some however
that are okay, these will be sweetened
with honey or just fruit and will use
butter or coconut oil, not vegetable oil
(more on this later).

Replacements- bake your own.
That way you can use minimal
sweeteners.

Breakfast Cereals

Contain up to a whopping 50%
sugar! If this is what you have for
breakfast, and find yourself going
through energy dips throughout the day,
now you know why. These need to be
avoided. Due to being processed at high
temperatures, all of the nutrients are
destroyed and as a result, the nutritional
benefits are depleted. Even the so-called
'healthy muesli/granola bars' are most
often ladened with sugar, as well as seed
oils.

Replacements- make your own soaked porridge or muesli instead. There are many other breakfast options that are much more nutritious and delicious, such as eggs and free range bacon or coconut flour pancakes.

Condiments

Such as ketchup, strawberry jam, salad dressings, mayonnaise, fruit chutneys and chocolate sauce are very high in sugar and usually contain additives. Even some nut butters need to be avoided as they often have sugar and vegetable oils added.

Replacements- natural nut butters, where the only ingredient is nuts. Pesto made with olive oil. Tomatoes instead of chutney and salsa, or better yet, fermented salsa. Berries instead of store bought jam, smash them up and serve on some bread, this is lovely on my paleo bread. Use olive oil with lemon juice or balsamic vinegar instead of store bought dressings or make your own mayonnaise.

Flavoured yoghurts

Are packed with sugar and additives.

29

Replacement- Natural full fat (greek) yoghurt with no sweeteners added. You can add your own fruit to sweeten or a small amount of rice malt syrup, raw honey or dark maple syrup.

Low-fat dairy products

Often have sugar added to replace the fat that has been removed and most of the nutrients are removed as well.

Replacements- Full fat dairy products

The following is a list of alternate names given to sugar. Be aware of these and know that they have the same affect on the body as table sugar. These names will be in the ingredient list and are a sneaky way of adding sugar.

• Barley malt	• Golden sugar
• Beet sugar	• Golden syrup
• Brown sugar	• Grape sugar
• Buttered syrup	• High-fructose corn syrup
• Cane juice crystals	• Honey
• Cane sugar	• Icing sugar
• Caramel	• Invert sugar
• Corn syrup	• Lactose
• Corn syrup solids	

• Confectioner's sugar	• Maltodextrin
• Carob syrup	• Maltose
• Castor sugar	• Malt syrup
• Date sugar	• Maple syrup
• Demerara sugar	• Agave syrup
• Dextran	• Molasses
• Dextrose	• Muscovado sugar
• Diastatic malt	• Panocha
• Diatase	• Raw sugar
• Ethyl maltol	• Refiner's syrup
• Fructose	• Sorbitol
• Fruit juice	• Sorghum syrup
• Fruit juice concentrate	• Sucrose
• Galactose	• Sugar
• Glucose	• Treacle
• Glucose solids	• Turbinado sugar
	• Yellow sugar

The truth is, we do not 'need' sugar in our diet at all, not even from fruit. The body can create the sugars we need from the rest of the food we consume. That is why you have never heard of an 'essential' sugar, like you have for fats and protein. You do not need to avoid fruit, but you should not be concerned if you do not eat it every day. When you eat traditional foods such as organic vegetables, pastured animal produce and full fat food items, you will supply your body with plenty of nutrients.

Cutting back on sugar may be difficult at times and it will take time for your body to adjust to the changes. However, you will stop 'needing' it and this will stop the cravings. Excess sugar in your diet may be the very reason you are not losing weight or why you get sick a lot. Keep this in mind and know that by reducing your sugar intake, you are creating a healthy body.

There may be times when you overindulge and have an excess amount of sugar. This is okay, do not beat yourself up, accept that it happened and move on. As your body is not used to the large quantity of sugar anymore, it will have a toxic effect on your system which can cause headaches and leave you feeling lethargic and just downright horrible. Listen closely to your body, it will tell you what it needs.

FUNDAMENTAL FATS

What first comes to mind when you hear the word fat?

is it;

A fatty substance made from animal or plant products, used in cooking

or

The presence of excess fat in a person or animal, causing them to appear corpulent.[16]

These are both definitions for the word fat but we tend to relate to the latter one. This is unfortunate because fat has numerous vital functions in the body. It is an essential part of your diet, you cannot live without it. It also brings so much flavour to a dish, making it enjoyable to eat.

We have become afraid of the word fat and are told to avoid it as much as possible, saturated fat in particular. Unfortunately this information is incorrect; fat is medicine for your body. Not only does it provide numerous health benefits, it keeps you satiated, thus you are less likely to overeat, avoiding weight gain and disease.

The story behind saturated fat being linked to heart disease and high cholesterol goes back to 1956 when a doctor named Dr. Ancel Keys conducted a study to ascertain if a diet high in saturated fats is linked to heart disease and high cholesterol. The problem is that he conducted the study on rabbits. As you know rabbits are herbivores, they are not designed to eat meat, so of course they are going to suffer if they consume saturated fats. Dr. Keys then went on to study the link with people. He studied twenty-two countries around the world with diets that were high in saturated fat hoping to correlate it with heart disease. Some had more saturated fat intake with less heart disease and others had less saturated fat intake with more heart disease, again his findings were inconclusive. Dr. Keys was looking to confirm his strong belief in his theory, he overlooked the data that contradicted his rabbit research, and selected the data that supported it. Basically, Dr. Keys chose just seven of the countries that fit his hypothesis and used these as evidence that saturated fat and high cholesterol did indeed cause heart disease. The amazing thing about Dr. Keys, is that he became important in the political arena, and his nutrition ideas went a great distance to lobby for a low fat diet in government. The evidence that saturated fat causes heart disease is flimsy to say the least, and lots of good research contraindicating this has been overlooked. For a great synopsis and review of this story see the book "Big Fat Lies: How the diet industry is making you sick, fat & poor" by David Gillespie. [17]

Fats, are vital to the proper functioning of the body. About half the energy used by the entire body at rest and during light activity, come from fat. Fats are also one of the main building blocks of every cell in your body. Fats are essential in maintaining healthy skin, and preventing premature ageing as well as the production of prostaglandins. Prostaglandins regulate body functions such as heart rate, blood pressure, blood clotting, fertility, conception, digestion and play a role in immune function by regulating inflammation and encouraging the body to fight infection. The fat soluble vitamins A, D, E, and K cannot be absorbed without fat present in the diet, and many other vitamins are better absorbed when eaten with fat.[18]

Types Of Dietary Fats

There are three broad categories of fatty acids; saturated fatty acids (SFA), monounsaturated fatty acids (MUFA) and polyunsaturated fatty acids (PUFA).[19] Foods containing fat are composed of all three types of fatty acids, however, there will be one type that is particularly high. For example, cheese is higher in saturated fatty acids, olive oil is higher in monounsaturated fatty acids and fish oil is higher in polyunsaturated fatty acids, but all foods contain all three types of fatty acids.

Saturated Fatty Acid: These fats tend to be solid at room temperature and due to their capabilities to withstand high heat, are the best choice for cooking. The best sources are from animals that live on green pastures and are not fed grain, at all. An exception is with chickens, they can tolerate grain, although it's best to avoid ones that are fed soy and any GMO's. It is vital that they have access to plenty of green pasture and grubs. Examples of good sources of saturated fatty acids include meat, eggs, milk, cheese, cream, yogurt, butter, lard and ghee. Coconut and cacao also provide a good source of saturated fatty acids. There are other sources of saturated fatty acids, but I recommend you consume the fats from the foods listed here.

Monounsaturated Fatty Acid: These fats are liquid at room temperature and semi solid or solid when refrigerated. They can withstand higher temperatures than polyunsaturated fats but they are not as stable as saturated fats. This allows them to be cooked at moderate heat. The best sources are from cold pressed extra virgin olive oil, cold pressed avocado oil and cold pressed nut oils.

Polyunsaturated Fatty Acid: These fats are liquid at room temperature and often stay liquid when refrigerated. They are the weakest of all the fatty acids at withstanding heat and as a result, become rancid easily.

Omega-6 and omega-3 are essential polyunsaturated fatty acids, meaning they cannot be made by the body and must be obtained in the diet. Sources come from plants such as nuts and seeds. However, these plant sources tend to have an unbalanced ratio of omega fatty acids, (apart from flax which has a higher omega- 3 to omega-6 ratio). The best sources come from cold pressed flaxseed oil, cold pressed marine oil such as cod liver oil, fatty fish such as salmon, and algae. You do not need to avoid nuts and seeds all together, but I suggest that these do not make up a large part of your diet. Remember that these contain phytic acid so it's best to consume ones that have been prepared correctly, meaning they have been soaked and dehydrated. You can prepare them at home by soaking the nuts in water with a little salt for twelve hours. Then either using a dehydrator or a low oven (around 76 degrees celsius) until the nuts are completely dried. Alternatively you can purchase activated nuts and seeds, these have already been through this process and are ready to eat.

Why You Need To Avoid Seed Oils

You may have heard polyunsaturated fatty acids named essential fatty acids (EFAs). They are essential to the body because we cannot make them and therefore, they must be obtained from food. There are two types of essential fatty acids, Omega-6 and Omega-3. Omega fats play an important role in the inflammatory cascade in our bodies. These fats are found in both plant and animal sources. Plant sources, however, provide an unbalanced ratio of omega-6 and omega-3 and this increases inflammation in the body. An excess amount of omega 6 in the diet without enough omega 3 is pro-inflammatory. The dietary ratio of omega-6 to omega-3 should be 1:1 or at most 2:1, anything outside this range can cause problems in the body. When omega-6 overwhelms the body, this causes inflammation and can lead to serious chronic conditions such as heart disease, cancer and depression.[20,21,22,23,24,25]

Unfortunately, today the average person consuming a western diet eats an omega-6 to omega-3 ratio of 16:1 and the typical diet today can contain up to thirty times more omega-6 to omega-3 fatty acids[26]. The cause of this unbalanced ratio is due to most fats coming from seed oils (vegetable oils). To allow for a greater shelf life, seed oils are hydrogenated. When vegetable oils are hydrogenated, their chemical structure is changed and even before you open the bottle, it is already rancid.[27]

In the 1990's scientist discovered the detrimental health effects that hydrogenated seed oils have on the body. These oils were causing heart disease, cancer, diabetes, arthritis, weight gain and obesity, hypertension and autoimmune disorders. [28]When researchers from the University of Maryland analysed data that was used to make claims that animal fat was linked to heart disease and cancer of various types, they found that vegetable fat in fact was the correlation and animal fat was not. These rancid oils are not only damaging your internal body, they also affect your appearance. By forming what is known as, reactive oxygen species (ROS) which damages the DNA/RNA (structure) of the body as well as the collagen in your skin. This damage has been linked to disorders from cancer to premature aging.[29]

I cannot emphasise the importance of eliminating these rancid seed oils from your diet enough, FOREVER. Such oils include corn, cottonseed, soybean, safflower and canola oils. I strongly suggest avoiding anything that has the ingredient 'vegetable oil' in it. Seed oils are hidden in pretty much all packaged foods such as, margarine, biscuits, cakes, potato chips, muesli/granola bars, fried foods, confectionary and some chocolate. Even so called 'healthy' food can contain seed oils, so be sure to check the ingredient list. When you are eating out, don't feel embarrassed to ask if the food contains seed oils, you are paying for it after all so you have the right to know exactly what you are eating. The best sources of polyunsaturated fatty acids come from whole nuts and seeds, wild caught fatty fish (salmon, mackerel, herring, sardines), flax seed oil, cod liver oil and fats from pastured animal produce.

When you avoid seed oils, you also stay away from Trans fats, a nasty by-product of hydrogenation of vegetable oils, the Food and Drug Administration (FDA) in the United States of America has just recently banned synthetic trans fats (there are some naturally occurring trans fats in most foods) and labeled them not fit for human consumption.[30]

The Truth About Animal Fats

You will have heard that saturated animal fats contribute to high cholesterol, heart disease and weight gain and I am troubled by this information because it is untrue.

A study conducted in 2010 and published in the American Journal of Clinical Nutrition, reviewed twenty-one studies on heart disease, stroke and saturated fats. They found that there is no significant evidence for concluding that dietary saturated fat is associated with an increased risk of CHD (coronary heart disease) or CVD (stroke and cardiovascular disease). [31] There have not actually been any studies that conclude fat causes heart disease and cutting down on the so called 'bad' fats has not helped the incidence of such diseases. In fact, they are still on the rise today but believe me, the consumption of saturated fats are not the reason.[32]

From 1910-1970, the proportion of traditional animal fat in the American diet declined from eighty-three percent to sixty-two percent, and butter consumption plummeted from 8.1 kilograms per person per year to 1.8 kilograms. During the same period the percentage of dietary vegetable oils in the form of margarine, shortening and refined oils increased about four hundred percent while consumption of sugar and processed foods increased about sixty percent. [33] If cutting back on saturated fats decreases heart disease, then why is it that even with the twenty one percent decrease in animal fats, forty percent of deaths in the US and thirty-three percent of deaths in Australia today are caused by heart disease? An important point to look at is the immense increase in refined vegetable oils and sugar that have replaced fats in the diet. The consumption of these have dramatically increased but have been ignored as a contributor to heart disease. With the increase in consumption of vegetable oils and sugar and the decrease in animal fats, also came a rise in weight gain and obesity levels.[34]

Animal products that have been grass-fed promote the following health benefits;[35,36,37]

- Improve bone health- saturated fat aids calcium absorption
- Lower Lp(a), a substance in the blood that indicates a propensity to heart disease.
- Protect the liver from toxins

- Enhance the immune system, maintain healthy skin and have antiviral and anti-fungal agents
- Help with utilisation of, and contain omega-3 fatty acids
- Have antimicrobial properties that help protect the digestive system
- Aid digestion and help with weight control and food cravings
- Regulate hormones
- Maintain cell structure
- Are crucial for absorbing vitamins
- Preventing heart disease, stroke and heart attack
- Reduce inflammation and may help to prevent arthritis

A VERY important factor to remember when choosing animal products is to make sure that they come from animals that live on pasture for their entire life. Produce can be labeled grass-fed but they are quite often finished on grain. Feeding grain causes the animal to gain weight (the same goes for us) which causes an unhealthy ratio of fats. Be sure to check that the animal produce you are buying has been one hundred percent grass-fed. Animals must be ethically raised on their natural diet, which is grass.

Compared to animals fed grain, pasture fed animals contain:

- Half the amount of fatty acids overall, meaning the ratio of fats is balanced
- Higher vitamin A and beta-carotene[38]
- Higher Conjugated linoleic acid (CLA), these are fatty acids that have cancer fighting properties and help with weight management. CLA helps to reduce body fat and increase lean muscle. Studies have shown that consuming 3.2g/day of CLA produced a significant ninety gram loss of fat and an increase of 1% lean muscle mass per week. Both of these results will contribute to raising the bodies metabolic rate, therefore burning more energy (calories). Of course this needs to be in conjunction with other aspects of a healthy lifestyle
- Higher omega-3s. Omega-3s are vital for growth and development, especially of the brain. This reason makes it vitally important that infants receive an adequate source of these super fatty acids. Just as important, are pregnant and breastfeeding women. Whatever the mother puts into her body directly works to nourish her baby. I cannot express enough, the fundamental importance of a diet that is filled with healthy saturated fatty acids whilst pregnant and breastfeeding[39]

Fats, saturated fats in particular, are needed to help with the absorption and utilisation of vitamins,

43

especially fat-soluble vitamins. Vitamins A and D help with calcium absorption and calcium cannot be utilised without vitamin D present, so getting some sun on your skin is important to build your vitamin D levels.

Choose Full Fat Dairy

To receive the nutritional benefits of dairy (that is if you are not sensitive to it of course), as well as enjoying the best flavour, it is best to choose full fat products from organic grass fed cows. Skim dairy products such as skinny (skim, 0% and 1%) milk and lite yoghurt, have been modified to suit the so-called 'healthy' low-fat diet. The fat has been removed from these products and as a result, they do not provide any nutritional benefits, nor do they taste pleasant. As vitamins A, D, E, & K are fat soluble, low-fat products do not supply these. These vitamins have numerous benefits from cell growth, healthy hair, skin and eyes to aiding absorption of phosphate and calcium. Calcium is lost during the making of skim dairy. As a result of this, it is replaced with synthetic calcium, which the body is not very effective at absorbing. To give these products body, powdered milk is often added and is usually not labeled on the list of ingredients. Powdered milk contains oxidised cholesterol which can lead to inflammation and plaque buildup in the arteries. Always choose full fat when purchasing all of your dairy produce. Enjoy the flavour that full fat provides, you will be very surprised about the difference in taste and how satisfying these foods are. Who could go past a bowl of strawberries with fresh cream or some homemade chocolate mousse!

Keep in mind that you need to make sure the dairy produce comes from grass-fed animals. I also strongly recommend when purchasing any animal produce that it is organic. Commercial produce is often fed an unnatural diet of grain, leading to the need for antibiotics. Hormones are also used to increase milk supply. Ingesting these is detrimental to your health.

Drink Raw Milk

It may worry you when you hear the words 'raw' and wonder if it is safe to drink. This is an interesting question, but have you ever thought why do we homogenise and pasteurise our food?

The reason pasteurisation of milk became popular was back in the late 1800's, cows began eating an unnatural diet of grain and were overcrowded in a poorly sanitised environments. These two factors lead to poor health of the cow and as a result, they produced unsanitary milk. To solve the problem it was concluded that milk needed to be pasteurised.

Pasteurising milk alters its natural form and it does not provide the same nutritional benefits. Milk that has been pasteurised has most of its nutrients stripped, Vitamin C is lost and twenty percent of iodine is destroyed. Phosphorous is destroyed making it very difficult for the body to absorb calcium that can cause low bone density contributing to osteoporosis.

Raw milk produced by grass-fed cows in a sanitary environment contains 120-150 different types of beneficial bacteria that work as a probiotic in the gut, which is great for immunity. Another benefit of unpasteurised milk is that the natural enzymes are not destroyed, including lactulose, which is responsible for the breakdown of lactose sugar in the milk. This enzyme is not present in pasteurised milk and may contribute to lactose intolerance. I have clients who suffer from lactose intolerance and are now drinking raw milk with no problems. Raw milk generally comes from grass-fed cows, it provides numerous benefits such as a healthy omega-3 to omega-6 ratio, high amounts of CLA which are cancer fighters and helps to build lean muscle and reduce fat. Like other milk, raw milk contains fat-soluble vitamins A, D, E and K however, these vitamins occur naturally and do not need to be added synthetically making them easy for the body to absorb. Drinking full fat milk is very important as it helps to absorb these vitamins.

Unfortunately it is illegal, in most areas, to sell raw milk, however, it is not impossible to find. There are small dairy farms that will sell it and you will find it at most farmers markets as well as some health food stores. It will be labelled something like 'Bath Milk'. Do some research for a supplier close by and make sure it is organic and comes from grass-fed animals.

I recommend that all dairy products be eaten raw, as much as possible. You can get some lovely cheeses that have not been pasteurised. Raw cream, butter and yoghurt are fantastic additions to a healthy kitchen. For further reading on raw milk see 'The Untold Story of Milk: Green Pastures, Contented Cows and Raw Dairy Products' by Ron Schmid.

Eat Organ Meats

Organ meats, also known as offal, consist of the liver, kidney, brain, heart and tripe and are the most nutrient dense part of the animal. In the past, organ meats were a normal part of the diet. At a young age, I remember my Mum telling me that, as a baby, she would feed me sheep's brains. Of course back then I cringed at the thought of eating 'brains' but now that I know the wonderful health benefits that organ meats provide, I have learned how to cook with them so that they are appetising, I incorporate them into my family's diet twice a week. Compared to muscle meat, organ meats have a much higher concentration of nutrients. They provide a good source of B vitamins as well as the fat soluble vitamins A, D, E and K. They also contain high amounts of essential fatty acids, including the important omega-3 fatty acids, EPA and DHA. They are also loaded with minerals such as, iron, potassium, calcium, sodium, magnesium, phosphorus, selenium, copper, iodine, zinc and manganese. Liver is the most concentrated source of vitamin A of any food. It is high in vitamin D and provides a great source of B12. Pâté is a delicious way of eating liver, it is lovely served with crackers. Pâté is a favourite of my husbands, he makes a batch for us to enjoy each week from organic, pastured chicken. You can get the recipe on my website. Other ways to incorporate organ meat into your meals is to add it, along with muscle meat, to casseroles. The flavour will be mild, and to be honest, I can not taste it at all. I like to add it to coconut curries. Another option, which I find to be really handy, is to kindly ask your meat supplier to grind some organ meats into a mince. I do this with beef, and then add the mince to ground beef and use it for burgers and meat sauces. Jasper loves organ meat. I often fry up a good size portion of the mince mix and freeze it in small amounts, making it a quick and easy meal. He happily scoops it up with his fingers and manages to get most of it into his mouth.

It may take a little time and experimenting cooking with organ meats, and to wrap your mind around eating them, but the health benefits certainly outweigh the effort. Be adventurous, you never know, they may become your new favourite food!

How To Cook With Fats

As you know, there are three different types of fatty acids; saturated fatty acids (SFAs), monounsaturated fatty acids (MUFAs) and polyunsaturated fatty acids (PUFA), which include the essential fatty acid (EFAs) omega-3 and omega-6. The less saturated the fatty acid is, the less stable it is, meaning the easier it is destroyed by light and heat. The more saturated the fatty acid is, the more sturdy it is and the higher its ability to withstand heat. Unsaturated fatty acids are very fragile and are damaged easily by heat and light causing them to spoil and become oxidised and rancid. To make sure that you do not spoil fat when cooking with it, you need to be aware of its smoke point. A smoke point is the temperature a fat can withstand before it becomes oxidised. As saturated fatty acids are more durable than unsaturated fatty acids, they have a higher smoke point, meaning that they can be cooked at higher temperatures. Storage is also important, keeping fatty acids, particularly unsaturated ones, in a dark cool place is important to prevent oxidation.

Saturated Fatty Acids

Butter, lard, tallow, ghee, and expeller pressed virgin coconut oil, are fantastic choices for cooking and frying and sautéing. Remember, when you buy animal produce, do make sure they are from pastured animals and are organic. Animal meat and coconut products are also a great source of short chain fatty acids which have been shown to help speed up metabolism and slow down cancer growth.

Monounsaturated Fatty Acids

Cold pressed olive, sesame, avocado, and walnut oil are great choices. These oils can withstand low to moderate heat and are best used once the dish is cooked, stir through after you have turned the stove off, or use them cold. Activated nuts and seeds (these are nuts and seeds that have been properly prepared) are also a great source of MUFAs.

Polyunsaturated Fatty Acids

Cold pressed flaxseed and cod liver oil are the best choices. These oils must not be cooked with. They have a very low smoke point and will oxidise easily. They are best taken as a supplement; personally, I do not like the taste of either oils and will take them by the spoonful followed by a sip of water. Some like the taste of flaxseed oil and drizzle it on their salad. As these oils spoil easily, do make sure that they are cold pressed and store them in a dark, cool place, I always keep mine in the fridge. Animal produce will provide some EFAs but oily fish contains high amounts.

A Word On Cholesterol

Cholesterol is a fundamental building block of all cells and is a healing agent to your body. It works to clear infection, heal wounds and remove free radicals caused by stress and toxins. It works as a team with saturated fat and the body cannot function without it. HDL (high-density lipoprotein) and LDL (low-density lipoprotein) have been labeled as the so called "good" and "bad" cholesterol, however these terms are imprecise. LDL and HDL are simply the proteins that carry cholesterol to and from tissues. For example, when the body suffers a wound, your endothelium (cell lining) is damaged. Endothelium is the squamous cell lining of all the capillaries and blood vessels in the body. The endothelium needs fat to repair itself (all the cell membranes of your body are made of fat). LDLs have the important job in carrying the cholesterol and fats to the site of damage so that repair can begin. Once the damage is restored the leftover cholesterol and fats are carried back to the liver by HDL. High levels of LDL is an indication of inflammation in the body. [40]

Think of Lipoprotein as a fire engine, Low Density Lipoprotein (LDL) is the fire engine as it leaves the fire station, full of water for the fire. It goes to the fire and empties the water (drops of cholesterol and fat) to put out the fire, then returns to the station. When it is returning it is lighter, and hence High Density Lipoprotein (remember, fat is lighter than water, and less dense, so the more fat, the lower the density). LDL and HDL are nonspecific markers for inflammation in the body. If you have a fever, your cholesterol will increase, if you have a burn or infection, your cholesterol will increase, if you have cancer, sometimes your cholesterol will increase, if you are dehydrated, your cholesterol can be high.

When your cholesterol is high, what needs to be evaluated is 'what is the body trying to repair?' and 'why does it need repairing?' Getting to the root of the cause is what is important and cholesterol plays a vital role in this by healing the body and restoring new cells.

Cholesterol has many other important functions such as;

- Plays a critical role in the structural integrity of every cell in your body
- Is a precursor to vital hormones such as testosterone, oestrogen, vitamin D and adrenalin
- Makes up bile salts which are important for digestion of fats and therefore play a role in the

proper function of the digestive system (your body uses about 1,000mg of cholesterol daily in your bile)[41]

- Helps to produce vitamin D. This is why foods containing vitamin D also contain cholesterol, as well as fat, these all work together. By limiting your cholesterol and fat consumption, you are also limiting your vitamin D stores. Cholesterol plays a role in synthesising vitamin D from sunlight, without it, vitamin D cannot be absorbed. Vitamins D is vital for the health of your bones and nervous system as well as mineral metabolism, insulin production, reproduction and immunity. It helps to regulate levels of calcium which contributes to the prevention of osteoporosis

- Acts as an antioxidant which helps protect against diseases such as cancer and heart disease

- Helps to maintain the health of the intestinal walls, a diet low in cholesterol can lead to leaky gut syndrome. Leaky gut syndrome is when there is damage to the intestinal lining which disrupts proper absorption of nutrients from food

- Low cholesterol has been linked to depression and aggressive behaviour this is due to the link that cholesterol has with the proper functioning of serotonin in the brain

- A breastfeeding mothers milk is made up of cholesterol and saturated fat (over 50% by dry weight). These are utterly vital in the development of the brain and nervous system of the baby

So Why Do Cholesterol Levels Rise?

As I mentioned earlier, cholesterol has a major role in dealing with the repair of damage throughout the body. When there is damage to the cells of the body, serum cholesterol levels increase as the cholesterol is transported to areas of distress. When there is damage to the arteries of the heart (atherosclerosis), cholesterol levels need to increase to repair the damage. Unfortunately this increased level of cholesterol has been associated with heart disease, but in fact, it is just simply the body's defence mechanism of repairing the damage in the arteries. What is also unfortunate is, foods that are high in saturated fatty acids, which are mostly animal products, are also high in cholesterol, they have been labeled as "bad" and have been warned that they should only make up a tiny proportion of the diet.[42]

Foods labeled 'lite' or 'fat-free' often contain hydrogenated fats, the hydrogenation process causes fats to become oxidised and do damage to the body. This is most often seen in foods containing refined carbohydrates, mostly seen in packaged foods and sweet baked treats. The consumption of excess refined carbohydrates leads to deficiencies in vitamin C, E and selenium. These are important antioxidants which play a role in clearing the body of free radicals, and as a result, cholesterol is needed for the healing process, and in turn the level of cholesterol in the blood increases.

Cholesterol is seen as the villain when it should be seen as the hero. It has a fundamental role in repairing damage in the body. The body is very good at making its own cholesterol, if it is running low, it will only produce more. When you eat foods that are high in cholesterol the body will decrease its cholesterol production. No matter how much you avoid eating foods containing cholesterol, your body will make what it needs anyway.[43] Dr Perlmutter makes a good point on the topic in his book 'Grain Brain'. *"We all make up to 2,000 milligrams of cholesterol every day because we desperately need it, and this is several times the amount found in our diets. But despite this amazing ability, it's critical to obtain cholesterol from dietary sources. Our bodies much prefer we 'spoon-feed' our cholesterol from our foods we eat rather than manufacture it internally, which is a complex multistep biological process that taxes the liver."*

In Summary

Your body is made up of saturated fat and cholesterol, so eating it is not bad for you. Look for fats from pastured animals, cold pressed or expeller pressed, virgin or extra virgin unrefined oils such as olive oil, coconut oil and cod liver oil. When choosing fats, it is extremely important to avoid refined vegetable seed oils such as soybean, sunflower, safflower and canola. These oils have often been hydrogenated turning them into trans fats which cause cancer, heart disease and obesity. Avoid consuming trans fats by avoiding margarine, vegetable shortening, cookies, cakes, potato chips, foods fried in vegetable oils, packaged and deep fried foods. It is just safer to stay away from any food product with "vegetable oil" as an ingredient.

PRIMARY PROTEIN

*A traditional food diet will contain all the
essential amino acids your body needs to thrive.*

Protein is crucial in the regulation and
maintenance of your body's functions and along with fat,
it helps to keep you full until your next meal.

Protein provides the following benefits; [44]

- repair and builds cells
- strengthens the immune system
- promotes normal growth, thus helps to build
  muscle
- forms hormones
- assists in blood clotting
- manufactures milk during lactation

All proteins are combinations of 22 amino acids,
8 of which are essential, meaning the body cannot make
them and they need to be obtained from the food we eat.
When all essential amino acids are present, the body can
build the other nonessential ones; but if just one essential
amino acid is missing, the body is unable to use the
other proteins it needs, even when protein intake is high.

Animal protein is the best source of complete
protein as all 22 amino acids are present. Plant protein

however, is incomplete, it is low in at least one of the essential amino acids. To get a complete supply of amino acids from plants, you need to ingest a mixture of different types of plant proteins. For example, legumes such as, peanuts, beans, cashews, lentils and peas contain the amino acid lysine but they are low in methionine. Grains such as, oats, rice, barley, corn and wheat contain the amino acid methionine but are low in lysine. To obtain complete protein from plant based foods, a mixture of both legumes and grains need to be consumed. The best way to make sure you get enough of both lysine and methionine is to combine legumes and grains in each meal. For example, toast with peanut butter or rice with lentils or spinach salad with sesame seeds. As plant based foods do not contain Vitamin B12 and Vitamin D and very little iron, zinc and calcium, vegetarians need to make sure that they get an adequate amount of eggs, dairy and sunlight to supply them with these nutrients and micronutrients. Also, if you are avoiding grains, eating plenty of these foods will provide protein. Some foods are fortified with vitamins, however the body does not absorb these synthetic vitamins well. Also, there are often other unnatural ingredients added which need to be avoided such as sugar, seed oils and preservatives.

Although protein plays a vital role in the body and is important to include, I believe that the amount of protein needed in the diet has been overemphasised.

High protein products seen on the market today such as protein powders and bars, are a waste of money and provide no health benefits. If you eat a traditional diet that contains animal fats, you will get more than enough protein to sustain and build a healthy body. Most people only need 0.7g to 1g of protein/kg of bodyweight per day and can easily reach this by eating traditional foods.

Summary Of Carbohydrates, Fats and Protein

Carbohydrates

- If you choose to include grains, avoid modern wheat and choose properly prepared, ancient grains instead, ideally gluten free.
- Limit fructose by avoiding packaged foods and bought baked goods. Do your own baking, that way you know exactly what is in it and can limit the amount of sugar
- The small amount of sugar consumed should come from whole fruits and small amounts of unrefined sweeteners
- Good sources of carbohydrates include properly prepared grains (if you eat them) such as quinoa, oats, brown rice and amaranth. If you choose a grain free diet- seasonal whole fruit and vegetables, nut and seeds (whole or as spreads and flours) are a good source. Also keep in mind

that you will get a small amount of carbohydrates from other food sources

Fats

- Include fats with each meal to be satiated
- Do not be afraid of saturated animal fats, remember all of those beneficial properties
- Consume organic grass-fed meat and eggs from pastured hens
- Avoid low-fat, no-fat and lite products
- Consume full fat dairy and find some raw milk
- Avoid rancid seed oils such as soy, canola, safflower and sunflower
- Get your EFAs from oily fish, animal produce, whole nuts and seeds and cod liver oil
- Store oils in a dark cool place to prevent oxidation and cook them gently
- Eat fat with vegetables so that you get your fat soluble vitamins, try butter or coconut oil
- Remember the benefits of cholesterol, the body creates its own so avoiding it is pointless and taxing on your liver
- Good sources of fat are full fat organic animal produce such as eggs, cheese, milk, yoghurt, cream, kefir and butter, activated nuts and seeds, extra virgin olive and sesame oil, expeller pressed virgin coconut oil, oily fish and cod liver oil

Protein

- Include protein with each meal to help you stay fuller for longer
- Consume protein with fat so that it is utilised efficiently
- Avoid protein supplements
- Animal protein is the best source of complete protein, here you will also get fat
- If you are getting your source from plants, remember you need to mix legumes with grains for it to be a complete protein, or make sure you eat plenty of dairy and eggs
- Good sources of protein are from animal produce such as meat, fish, eggs and dairy. You can also get protein in plant sources such as nuts and legumes but it is not as high

METABOLISM, YOUR POWER HOUSE

Metabolism: The sum of the processes in the buildup and destruction of protoplasm; specifically : the chemical changes in living cells by which energy is provided for vital processes and activities and new material is assimilated.[45]

Metabolism is the amount of energy in the form of calories that your body burns to maintain a specific disequilibrium. The body is constantly burning calories to supply you with energy to get you through everyday activities. These calories are needed for proper functioning of internal organs. Without sufficient calories, your organs will be compromised. Whether you are eating, sleeping, digesting food, or sitting on the couch, your metabolism is continually running. Metabolism is the disequilibrium of life.

Depriving the body of calories to lose weight can actually have the opposite effect. The body will think it is starving and as a defence, it will store fat for future use. If losing weight is a goal of yours, you need to make sure you provide your body with sufficient calories so that it can function efficiently. Fat burning is part of a normal healthy metabolism.

Being aware of the factors that affect your metabolism will give it the best chance to function well. Such factors include:

- Body composition- your muscle to fat ratio affects the speed of your metabolism. Muscle uses more energy than fat therefore, the more muscle you have, the faster your metabolism will be
- Genetics- your genetic makeup governs the speed of your metabolism
- Sleep- sleep plays a vital role in regulating metabolism. If you are not getting enough, it causes an imbalance in your metabolic system. The hormones leptin and ghrelin are disrupted and these are important in appetite control. Sleep deprivation interferes with your mood and as a result, you are more likely to make poor food choices, usually filling up on simple carbohydrates. It is important to go to bed at a reasonable hour and try to get at least seven hours of sleep per night
- Age- during your 20's your metabolism will begin to slow down and once you reach your 30's you will begin to lose muscle mass which also slows metabolism. This is the normal process of the body and it just means that you require less energy and therefore less food as you get older

- Resting Metabolic Rate (RMR)- this is much the same as your base metabolic rate (BMR). Your RMR is the rate at which your body burns calories when it is resting. This accounts for around 65-75% of your total daily calorie expenditure. For your metabolism to function effectively, you need to make sure that you fuel it with enough food to meet your RMR. As I mentioned earlier, if you deprive your body of calories, your metabolism will slow down to survive. This survival mode will cause you to store fat and gain weight
- Food Supply- the amount of time left between meals. If you like to eat large meals, (making sure it has a sufficient amount of fat) you will stay full and be able to go longer between meals. If you prefer a smaller meal, you may like to have a snack in between, just be sure that the snacks are nutrient dense. If you find that you cannot control how much you snack, eating larger meals, less frequently may suit you better
- Exercise- your metabolism does speed up during exercise and for a little time after. Exercise will also help to build muscle, contributing to a more active metabolism

You will have seen numerous products that claim to increase your metabolism on the market today but I suggest that you avoid such products. Your metabolism is an innate bodily function and really does not require much to do its job. Getting sufficient sleep, eating a balanced diet containing traditional, nutrient rich foods and exercising regularly will allow your metabolism to function efficiently, contributing to your overall health and wellbeing.

WONDERFUL WATER

The body is made up of around seventy-two percent water. Being properly hydrated will contribute to the proper functioning of the body. The brain cannot function well if you are dehydrated and can lead to loss of concentration and even headaches or migraines.

Other important functions of water are:

- Transport nutrients and oxygen into your cells as well as aiding the absorption of nutrients
- Protect vital organs
- Regulate body temperature
- Protect and lubricate your joints
- Maintain metabolism
- Aid proper functioning of your kidneys which helps to detoxify your body by helping to eliminate waste
- Hydrate and nourish your skin
- Keeps your digestion regular
- Prevents overeating- sometimes you may think that you are hungry but really you are dehydrated. Therefore, staying hydrated plays a role in maintaining and losing weight

Harmful effects dehydration has on your body are:

- Irregular blood pressure

- Constipation
- Dry skin, keeping your skin hydrated helps to prevent premature aging
- Tiredness and fatigue
- Headaches and migraines
- Muscle cramps
- Kidney problems
- Poor concentration
- Moodiness

Symptoms of dehydration are:

- Dark urine- when you are well hydrated your urine should be pale yellow or clear in colour
- Dry skin
- Thirst- this means that you are already dehydrated
- Hunger
- Fatigue and feeling unwell in general

Water plays numerous vital roles in your body and prevents many unpleasant symptoms. So how much do you need for your body to function properly? As your are constantly losing water you need to make sure you replace it with a sufficient amount. One litre per 25 kilogram of body weight per day is a good guide to go by (to work out how many litres you need simply divide your body weight in kg by 25 (by 56 if your weight is in pounds). If there are other activities in your life that cause you to lose extra fluid, such as intense exercise or hot days, you will need to drink more. A great way to know that you are well hydrated is to check the colour of your urine, remember it needs to be pale yellow to clear in colour and should have no odour.

If you know that you are not drinking enough water each day and need to increase it, at first this can be a little difficult, as your body is not used to drinking a large amount. I recommend introducing the extra water slowly, for example, drink 100 ml extra each day until you have reached your ideal consumption.

If you struggle to drink water because you do not like the taste, you can add natural flavours to make it more pleasant, such as sliced fruit, a squeeze of citrus juice, essential oils or dilute your favourite tea. When you start to drink more water, you will adjust to the taste and it will become easy for you to consume your recommended amount. Filtered water also taste a lot better so purchasing yourself a filter water jug or bottle is a great investment. Also, be sure to use glass or Bisphenol A (BPA) free bottles to prevent you from consuming the harmful toxins. Avoid purchasing water in plastic bottles as much as possible as they are not BPA free. BPA is an industrial chemical that has been used to make certain plastics and resins since the 1960s. Some research shows that storing food and beverages in containers containing BPA can allow the BPA to leach into the food and beverage which can pose health risk on the brain, behaviour and prostate gland of foetuses, infants and children. It is best to avoid BPA as much as possible.[46,47]

CALORIE COUNTING IS HISTORY

Forget counting calories, enjoy good quality, nutrient rich food and build the body of your dreams.

For many years now, we have been told that in order to lose weight, we need to restrict calorie intake. Numerous "diets" call for calorie counting and have you eating fewer calories than your body requires to function on a day to day basis. This leaves you feeling deprived and ravenously hungry; in general, you tend to feel unhappy about life. Consider this the last time you counted calories, it is a tedious task and its results do not last. Food nourishes your body, it is not your enemy, it should be enjoyed, so learn to love it back.

It is true that if you eat more calories than you burn, you are likely to gain weight however, calories from different sources (carbohydrates, fats and protein) affect your body differently, and this makes a huge difference in maintaining and losing weight.

What is a calorie?

A calorie is a measure of energy derived from a food source. [48] Each macronutrient has a measure of calories per gram. A gram of fat has nine calories and a gram of both protein and carbohydrates have four. Fat has more than double the amount of calories per gram.

When the food industry use calorie counting as a guide to losing weight fat is generally restricted due to its higher calorie levels per gram but this theory does not work. The body is designed to survive, if you restrict food intake, and fat in particular, it will defend itself by storing fat to survive and, as a result, you will not be able to shift weight. Another problem with using calories as a guide to losing weight is that the body metabolises fats, carbohydrates and protein differently, making the measurements inaccurate.

A study published in The Journal of the American Medical Association (JAMA) found that people on a low-carbohydrate/higher fat and low GI (which was also lower carbs and higher fat but not as low as the low-carb diet) burned more calories through the day compared to those on a low-fat/high carbohydrate diet. For weight loss and maintaining weight, the low GI diet is said to be most beneficial as it is easier to stick to and much healthier for the body. This translates to lasting results. This diet has 40% of calories coming from fats, 40% coming from carbohydrates (all from complex carbohydrates) and 20% coming from protein.[49]

Depriving your body of any of the important macronutrients makes it very difficult to lose and maintain weight. It is also harmful to the body as it prevents the consumption of essential nutrients and the

71

deprivation leads to a very unpleasant way of living. Again, the presence of fat and limited amount of simple carbohydrates has proven to be important factors in overall health, both on the inside and out. You must really be seeing the vital importance fat plays in your body now.

A Few Tips For Losing Weight

Along with what you have learned so far in my book, here are a few tips for losing weight:

- Forget calorie counting- rather than focusing on the amount of calories, focus on the quality of food you get them from, this will generate the best results.

- Eat foods that are higher in fat and lower in carbohydrates- feeling full will give you the best chance to lose and maintain weight, and one of the ways to do this is to eat more fat and less carbohydrates. Do not cut out carbohydrates, just make sure that your calories come from foods that are higher in fat (which will also be higher in protein) this way, you will be eating less carbohydrates. Remember, providing your body with an adequate supply of fats, and saturated fats in particular, (such as coconut oil, butter, cream, milk, meat and eggs), produces the hormone to tell your brain that you are full. Fats will prevent food binges because you will be satiated, you will not feel hungry which will help to curb your cravings.

- Eat coconut oil every day- the medium chain fatty acids (MCFAs) found in coconut oil stimulates weight loss by boosting the metabolism. It also helps with proper thyroid function. When the thyroid is functioning well, weight loss is accelerated.

EATING ORGANIC

Many years ago organic food did not exist. Food was naturally free of harmful pesticides, hormones and antibiotics, and therefore, all food was what is today considered organic. Traditional farming methods used crop rotation, intercropping and livestock to control pests. The plants were rotated in a way to increase soil nutrients, and the animals ate what they were designed to eat. This is not the fact in modern day production methods.

What is organic farming?

The word "organic" refers to the way farmers grow and process agricultural products, such as fruits, vegetables, grains, dairy products and meat. Organic farming practices are designed to encourage soil and water conservation and reduce pollution. Farmers who grow organic produce do not use conventional methods to fertilise, control weeds or prevent livestock disease, they use only natural occurring chemicals or traditional remedies. For example, rather than using chemical weed killers, organic farmers conduct more sophisticated crop rotations and spread mulch or manure to keep weeds at bay. Instead of using antibiotics and growth hormones in animals, preventative measures are used such as paddock rotation. This allows the stock to roam outside on their natural diet which is pasture, they are feed a balanced organic diet and are kept in clean housing.

What are the health risks with consuming pesticides, hormones and antibiotics?

Fruit and vegetables are sprayed with chemicals to keep the pests from destroying the produce. This allows for greater shelf life and transportation to the supermarket and then 'freshness' in your home for a few days. The problem with this is the longer a fruit or vegetable sits after it has been picked, the less nutritious it is. Also, the produce is often picked too early, before the full flavour has developed, leaving them tasteless.

Consuming food that is treated with pesticides poses many health risks, including increased risk of cancer, birth defects, infertility, miscarriages and a weakened immune system.[50,51,52] Hormones are used in meat and dairy to increase the production of milk and the mass of the beast. Consuming foods containing these hormones have been linked to an increase risk of cancer and hormonal disruptions.

Antibiotics are routinely fed to livestock, poultry, and fish on industrial farms to promote faster growth and to compensate for the unsanitary conditions in which they are raised. Consuming produce containing this exposes your body to small amounts of antibiotics. Over time, this can disrupt the body's bacterial biome which can lead to improper function of your immune system. Organically farmed animals are raised in a sanitary environment where disease is less of a concern. Basically healthy animals raised on natural foods with enough space do not get sick as often as animals that are fed improper food and housed too densely.

Tips on eating organic:

Try your best to eat organic as much as possible, especially fruit and vegetables that are eaten whole, meaning you consume the skin and flesh. For example: broccoli, spinach, tomatoes, beans, apples, pears, peaches and berries. Foods that can be on your 'not as important' list are ones where the skin will not be eaten such as, avocados, pineapples and bananas. I strongly recommend that all animal produce be organic.

One of the best places to buy your produce is from farmers markets. You will be supporting your local farmers and be able to purchase fantastic fresh produce. You also have the opportunity to ask the farmer what they use to control pests and disease and therefore, will know if their produce is acceptable to you. These markets tend to be cheaper than health food stores and supermarkets, I even find them cheaper than non organic supermarket produce at times.

Making the change to organic eating can seem daunting and costly at first but prioritising the health of your family is what is most important. Perhaps you could replace an item that you consider not so necessary for an organic option; a great choice would be packaged food. Making swaps like this will allow you to slowly create an organic home.

Eating 100% organic is ideal however this does not have to happen right away, you can make the changes slowly. Think of it as though you are weaning yourself off non-organic food by prioritising food groups. The following is a list of most important to less important foods eaten organically; animal produce, fruit and vegetables consumed with the skin, fruit and vegetables consumed without the skin, nuts and seeds and baked goods.

You want to nourish your body and build immunity so that you have the energy to enjoy your life. Traditional organic food will provide you with that nutrition, without all the nasty chemicals from industrial food.

SOY AND ITS DANGERS

Unfermented soy products pose numerous health risks and they need to be avoided. The United Kingdom's chief medical officer and the British Dietetic Association concluded that the proven risks of soy outweigh the possible benefits.

What are the told benefits of soy?

- Soy is said to alleviate menopausal symptoms however, this statement has been found to be inconsistent.
- It provides protein, calcium, iron and zinc however unfermented soy also contains phytic acid which binds these minerals making them unavailable to the body.
- Soy claims to be healthy due to its low cholesterol levels, but you now know all about cholesterol and know that the 'low cholesterol diet' being healthy is nonsense.

So why is soy so bad?[53,54,55]

- Soy contains phytoestrogens, a group of plant-based oestrogen that mimic the natural oestrogen in the body. The consumption of these oestrogens disrupts endocrine function and has been linked to breast cancer, hormonal imbalances, early onset of puberty and both male and female infertility.

- Phytoestrogens are potent antithyroid agents that cause hypothyroidism and may cause thyroid cancer. Improper functioning of the thyroid can lead to difficulties losing and maintaining weight.
- Vitamin B12 in soy is not absorbed and actually increases the body's requirement for it.
- Soy increases the body's requirement for vitamin D.
- Soy causes disruptions in the menstrual cycle. Drinking just two glasses of soy milk daily for one month has enough phytoestrogens to alter a menstrual cycle.
- Pregnant women need to be aware that eating soy can be detrimental to their baby as it disrupts the hormonal development. Also, soy may be the reason, or contribute to difficulties with falling pregnant.
- Soy has harmful effects on infants who are fed a soy formula. It has been estimated that infants who are exclusively fed soy formula receive the equivalent of five birth control pills worth of oestrogen every day.
- There have been links to autoimmune thyroid disease.
- Soy weakens the immune system

- Soy is one of the top eight most common food allergens making you at risk of suffering an allergic reaction.
- There is a relationship with soy formula consumption and the development of ADHD and behavioural problems in children.

Not all soy products need to be avoided

Fermented soy products such as tempeh, natto, miso, tamari, and unpasteurised soy sauce are actually products that are good for you. This is due to the fermentation process that makes the availability of isoflavones greater which is associated with cancer prevention. It also encourages the friendly bacteria in the large intestine, which neutralises the unfriendly bacteria and allows for greater general assimilation of foods and nutrients.

The soy products to avoid are soy-milk, bean curd, tofu (almost all tofu is not fermented), soy flour, soy protein powder, soy infant formula, soy meat alternatives (these are most often made from hydrolysed soy powder), soy oil, soy lecithin (this is in almost every packaged food), textured vegetable protein (TVP), hydrolysed vegetable proteins or vegetable oils. These have been genetically engineered and are not in their organic form like fermented soy products, making them harmful to the body.

SUPER OILS

There are two oils which I call 'super oils'. Both of them provide immense health benefits and I strongly recommend including them in your daily diet.

Cod Liver Oil

Cod liver oil began showing up in the fishing communities of Norway, Scotland, and Iceland in the middle of the nineteenth century. During times of illness, the fisherman used cod liver oil because they had learned over the years that its medicinal properties were a natural, effective remedy for many of the infections that they developed.

Why is this super oil so good for you?

Cod liver oil contains large amounts of the omega-3 fatty acids DHA and EPA and preformed vitamin A and vitamin D. These are essential nutrients that are difficult to obtain in sufficient amounts through diet. EPA acts as the precursor of important prostaglandins which are localised tissue hormones that help the body deal with inflammation. DHA is extremely important for the development and function and maintenance of the brain and nervous system.[56]

Cod liver oil also provides the following health benefits:

- Reduces and fights inflammation. This helps to prevent illness and disease such as heart disease and stroke and can also help to relieve arthritis
- Improves brain function and memory and can help to improve learning and behavioural disorders
- Decreases stress
- Fights infections by strengthening the immune system
- Helps to prevent allergies and asthma
- Builds healthy skin and hair
- Strengthens bones
- Improves the cell membrane for better nutrient absorption and toxin release
- Due to the source of vitamin D, calcium and magnesium are better absorbed which helps to lower blood pressure
- Provides protective properties against cancer

How much cod liver oil should you take?

I advise that you take one tablespoon of cod liver oil for adults and one teaspoon for infants and children most days of the week. Due to the flavour of the oil, you may find it difficult to take. Personally, I take the oil on a teaspoon and then immediately have a drink of water. The taste will not last longer than a few seconds, I promise. Otherwise, you can buy it with lemon flavouring, this takes away quite a lot of the liver flavour.

When purchasing cod liver oil, be sure to choose a brand that has been cold expressed as the fatty acids can be destroyed easily. This oil contains mainly PUFAs and must be stored in the fridge to avoid spoilage.

Coconut Oil [57]

Coconut oil contains a high proportion of saturated fatty acids that makes it very stable and can be cooked at high temperatures without oxidation. The very reason coconut oil was used in baked goods and packaged foods in the nineteenth century, as the oil can remain stable, preventing rancidity and health problems. During the middle of the twentieth century, coconut oil was used less and was replaced by hydrogenated vegetable oils. Just like animal fats, coconut oil consumption decreased due to the idea that saturated fat causes heart disease, but you now know that idea is just a myth, and like animals fats, coconut oil provides numerous benefits.[58]

The flesh of the coconut is very nutritious containing fibre, fat, calcium, magnesium, zinc, iron, potassium and vitamins B, C and E. All coconut products provide amazing health benefits and are fantastic for cooking and baking. Try using coconut cream in casseroles, coconut milk in smoothies and baked goods or desiccated coconut on top of yoghurt. Try my 'Chocolate Coconut Slice' or 'Little Chocolate Puddings' Always choose full fat varieties and avoid brands with added ingredients.

As coconut oil is mostly composed of saturated fats, it is solid at room temperature and begins to soften at twenty-four degrees Celsius. There are a few methods of producing coconut oil:[59]

1) Wet Milling- this is when the coconut flesh is shredded and cold pressed whilst moist. The meat, milk and oil are then fermented for at least 24 hours so that the water and oil can separate. The oil is then gently heated so that moisture can be removed and the oil can be filtered.

2) Expeller Pressed- in this process, the oil is made with a screw-like machine that squeezes the oil from the coconut meat. By using high pressure and friction to force coconut flesh through a caged barrel, expeller machines can extract up to 75 percent of the coconuts natural oil.

3) Industrial Coconut Oil- this type of oil is made by extracting oil from the copra (dried

coconut meat). To make it edible, the oil is refined, bleached and deodorised which destroys vitamins and flavour. Clearly, this type of oil needs to be avoided.

Coconut oil provides the following health benefits;

- Boosts Immunity

    Coconut oils main fat is 'lauric acid'. This has antibacterial, anti-fungal and antiviral properties which help to strengthen the immune system by fighting against viruses, bacteria and other pathogens.

- Helps Weight Loss

    The medium chain fatty acids (MCFAs) found in coconut oil require extra energy to be metabolised. The body's temperature increases which demands more calories and raises metabolic rate. This process aids weight loss. A study published in the American Journal of Clinical Nutrition, 1991, found that humans consuming a meal containing 30 grams (2 tablespoons) of MCFAs and 8 grams (about 1.5 teaspoons) of LCFAs had a significant rise in temperature compared to those who ate the same meal containing 38 grams of LCFAs. This rise in temperature indicates higher metabolic activity caused by increased thyroid functioning. Coconut oil helps your thyroid and boosts your metabolism.

- Prevents Heart Disease

  Virgin coconut oil has been found to prevent LDL-oxidation. Oxidised cholesterol can initiate the process of atherosclerosis, the fatty acids in coconut oil prevent this oxidation and therefore help to prevent heart disease. Studies dating back to the 1930s show that South Pacific Islanders whose diets were high in coconut oil were virtually free of heart disease. [60]

- Aids Skin Health

  Coconut oil can be used as a body and face moisturiser and is marvellous for keeping the skin soft and supple. I mix it 50/50 with jojoba oil, it absorbs into the skin really well. Coconut oil is fantastic for babies and children. It is antibacterial, anti-fungal and antiviral properties help to keep the skin clean, making it great to use on scrapes and cuts. It is great alternative to nappy cream (this is the

only product that I have used on Jasper),
a chemical free way to prevent nappy
rash.[61]

- Fantastic For Cooking

  Coconut oil is mainly saturated
  fats and it has a high smoke point making
  it perfect for cooking with. Try it in stir-
  fries, baked goods, casseroles and curry.
  Fried eggs in coconut oil are delicious. [62]

How much coconut oil should you take?

Two to three tablespoons a day will provide you
with wonderful benefits. It can be taken by the spoonful,
I don't actually like this so I in-cooperate it in my baking
and cooking.

Essential fatty acids (found mainly in cod liver
oil) can not be effectively assimilated and stored in the
tissues without the presence of adequate saturated fatty
acids. Therefore, it is great to take cod liver oil and
coconut oil together.

VITAMINS- GET THEM FROM REAL FOOD

Vitamins are essential nutrients that perform specific and vital functions in a variety of your body's systems, they are crucial for maintaining optimal health and keeping your immune system strong allowing you to take on each day with optimal energy. Your body uses thirteen vitamins. Not surprisingly, twelve of these can be found in meat.

Water Soluble Vitamins

The eight B group vitamins and Vitamin C are all water-soluble vitamins. The body needs water-soluble vitamins frequently but in small amounts, as they cannot be stored in the body. Water-soluble vitamins travel freely through the body, and excess amounts are usually excreted by the kidneys in your urine. Water-soluble vitamins act as coenzymes that help the body obtain energy from food. They are also important for normal appetite, good vision, healthy skin, nervous system function, and red blood cell formation as well as strengthening the immune system and building collagen.

Fat Soluble Vitamins

Vitamins A, D, E and K are fat-soluble vitamins. Fat-soluble vitamins are stored in the liver and fat (adipose) tissues. Due to this, they do not need to be consumed as frequently yet adequate amounts are needed. Fat soluble vitamins are important in providing adequate growth, building immunity, aiding absorption of other vitamins, assisting in blood clotting, acting as antioxidants to reduce free radical damage and are vital for bone, reproductive and skin health. As fat-soluble vitamins are stored in liver and tissue fat, they are not excreted quickly like water-soluble vitamins. Taking this type of vitamins in supplement form can lead to a greater chance of vitamin toxicity and can be harmful to the liver.

Are Synthetic Vitamins Necessary?

Billions of dollars are spent on vitamin supplements each year. It is great that we are trying to take control of our health but synthetic vitamins and minerals are not the best choice. Synthetic supplements, in my opinion, are a waste of money and in fact can be dangerous if taken in excess. A diet consisting of traditional foods makes synthetic supplements unnecessary. You can easily obtain an adequate amount of both water and fat-soluble vitamins by including the following foods in your diet each day:

- at least four cups of seasonal vegetables, served with butter or coconut oil and a sprinkle of himalayan rock salt
- Up to three servings of seasonal fruit. Berries are a great choice as they are high in antioxidants and lower in fructose compared to other fruit. If you do not want fruit, just make sure to eat more vegetables.
- Pastured, organic meat and wild caught fish (50-100 grams, depending on your size). If you are a vegetarian make sure you include dairy and eggs (if tolerated) so that you get a sufficient amount of fat and protein.
- Include organic eggs from pastured hens, if tolerated, organic dairy (raw if possible) such as full fat, grass-fed milk, cheese, yoghurt and butter as well as a small amount of nuts, seeds and nut butters.
- To get vitamin D, take cod liver oil and expose your whole body to the sun. Fifteen minutes a day is enough time to get a sufficient amount of vitamin D. This can be difficult in the winter months so make the most of it when the sun is shining. Be sure to leave the sun block off though, otherwise it will defeat the purpose. Try to go out when the sun is not at peak to avoid getting sun burnt.

Circumstances When Supplements May Be Necessary

- Vegetarians and vegans- need to keep in mind that as vitamin B12 can only be obtained in animal produce a supplement is more than likely necessary, unless an adequate amount of eggs and dairy are consumed.
- Pregnant, breastfeeding and women who are planning on becoming pregnant- It is a good idea that these women take a pregnancy vitamin, I strongly recommend to begin taking it at least three months before conception. This is mainly to get a sufficient amount of folate. It is important to choose a brand containing 'folate' and not folic acid as folate is metabolised better by the body.

When you are cooking your food, keep in mind that water-soluble vitamins are easily destroyed, especially vitamin C, try to lightly steam your vegetables. Eat them al dente and have a mix of both cooked and raw. Cooking in boiling water, or using the microwave, will destroy more vitamins than streaming.

WHAT TO DO WHEN YOU ARE FEELING RUN DOWN

A traditional diet helps to build a strong immune system. This will provide you with energy and help to lessen the risk of developing a cold or flu. However, there may be times when your immune system becomes weak and needs a little help recovering to its full strength. As soon as there are any signs of feeling unwell, be sure to stay well hydrated, get adequate sleep, relax and most importantly consume foods that will boost your immune system.

The key to avoiding a full blown cold or flu is to address the symptoms as soon as possible. The best way to do this is to rest and consume a range of traditional foods. The following are tips on what to do when you feel that cold coming on.

- Vitamins A, C, D, E, selenium and zinc all play a role in strengthening the immune system. Include foods that are high in these such as any organic pastured/grass-fed animal produce (especially eggs for the vitamin A and selenium), wild caught oily fish, cod liver oil, nuts (especially brazil nuts), fresh organic vegetables, especially sweet potatoes and carrots for the vitamin A (be sure to serve them with butter or coconut oil) getting sunlight will give you a good supply of vitamin D.

- Avoid sugar- just thirty grams of sugar is enough to suppress your immune system. This is the time to choose fruit (but not too much) over any other sweetener, as it will provide you with vitamins and minerals. Choose berries or citrus as they are higher in vitamin C.
- Saturated fats from organic pastured animals, coconut oil and other coconut products and mushrooms- these all have antibacterial and anti-fungal properties.
- Protein- this will help to re-build any damaged cells.
- Fermented foods- these are probiotics and have beneficial bacteria which will help to fight bacteria and viruses. Yogurt, raw milk, cheese, kombucha, sauerkraut and other fermented condiments are all fantastic choices.
- Bone broth- this is high in minerals and calcium and is a great way to make a hearty soup.
- Antioxidant rich foods- these will help to fight free radicals that do damage to your cells. Include foods such as organic berries (blueberries have the most), organic red peppers, tomatoes, kale, spinach, broccoli, kidney beans and green tea.

- Garlic, ginger, chilli and turmeric- these have anti-inflammatory properties as well as bacterial, viral and fungal fighting properties.
- Water- this will help to keep you hydrated and flush any toxins from your body.
- Sleep- you need to make sure that you get sufficient sleep. This will help your body to repair, get at least eight hours but sleep for as long as you can.
- Stress less- stress is not good at any time in your life and especially when your body is fighting off a cold. Take some time to relax, lie on the couch and read a book, watch a movie or take a long hot bath.
- Move- it is important to rest but it is also good to move your body a little too. This could just be some stretches or a short walk to get some fresh air and some vitamin D at the same time.

FERMENTED FOODS & BEVERAGES

Fermentation : An enzymatically controlled anaerobic breakdown of an energy-rich compound (as a carbohydrate to carbon dioxide and alcohol or to an organic acid); broadly : an enzymatically controlled transformation of an organic compound[63]

Fermented foods and beverages are very much apart of a traditional diet. Fermentation is used by many cultures around the world. It is a technique that is praised for its healing properties. This entails consuming fermented foods and beverages each day which enables the body to build beneficial bacteria that help it to thrive.

Your body contains bacteria, yeast, fungi and viruses. In fact, there are at least one hundred times more of these critters than you have cells, we are a symbiotic community of organisms. If these microbes are balanced, they are able to efficiently heal the body but an imbalance of these microbes can lead to disease. Nowadays we are afraid of germs, we over sanitise by washing and sterilising, thinking that this will keep us from getting sick. When we do become sick, we take antibiotics which further throws our microbes off balance. We are destroying these beneficial symbionts and our body is suffering as a consequence. We are also no longer consuming food that provide probiotics and enzymes. Raw dairy has been replaced by pasteurised products which destroys these enzymes. We no longer consume traditional lacto-fermented versions of sauerkraut and pickles and fermented beverages have been replaced by sugar ladened sodas.

So how do we acquire these beneficial bacteria?

Fermented foods go through a lacto-fermentation process. During this process, natural bacteria feed on sugar and starch creating lactic acid which preserves the foods nutrients and allows for better digestion. This process produces various strains of probiotics as well as beneficial enzymes, omega-3 fatty acids and vitamins. Fermented foods and beverages will introduce beneficial bacteria into the digestive system, which in turn, provides a correct balance of bacteria. This will help to improve bowel health, slow some disease, aid digestion and improve immunity. Proper balance of bacteria and enough digestive enzymes in the gut allows for efficient absorption of nutrients from food. If your body is able to absorb the nutrients supplied by foods, there is no need for supplements and synthetic vitamins, it will take all it needs from the traditional nutrient rich foods.

What are fermented foods and beverages?

Fermented foods and beverages can be easily prepared in the comfort of your own home and are extremely cost effective. These products are beginning to become popular and are available in health food stores and farmers market which is great to see.

Fermented beverages include kombucha, water, coconut and milk kefir, kvass and original ginger beer. Fermented foods include sauerkraut, raw dairy such as yoghurt, cheese and milk, creme fraiche, fermented pickles, lacto-fermented salsa and chutneys, lacto-fermented vegetables, kimchi and fermented soy such as miso and tempeh.

Soaking foods in water is also a form of fermentation. Soaking a bean, grain, or seed in water causes the outer hull to be broken down by probiotics which enables the sprouting process. Foods treated in this way have higher, more easily absorbed nutrient content. Sprouting also reduces the content of anti-nutrients, such as phytic acid, which inhibits the absorption of minerals such as iron and zinc from these grains.

EXERCISE, FIND YOUR PASSION

The exercise choice you make will have an impact not only on your health but also your happiness!

Including exercise into your everyday life is important. It helps to build strong bones, strengthen and tone muscles and prevent disease. It is great at boosting your mood and increasing your energy. There are many reasons that exercise is good for your health, these are just a few.

Exercise does help with maintaining and losing weight, however, I think that there is too much emphasis placed on this. We no longer exercise for fun, we exercise so that we do not become fat, and this is where the war against our body begins.

Have there been days where you have not felt like exercising? Perhaps this is everyday? Exercising because you enjoy the exercise of your choice means that you are much more likely to continue doing it. If you are exercising to lose weight, this may mean that you will find it very hard to get motivated and exercise may always be a struggle for you. Many years ago, the gym was my choice of exercise. I would get up each day, unmotivated to exercise, but I knew that I 'had' to if I wanted to achieve the body I was after. So I would put on my workout clothes and make my way to the gym, jump on a few machines and watch the clock, the entire time. It drove me crazy! I hated working out but I did not think I had any other choice. Until I explored my options, and then I found yoga. I initially started yoga because I thought it would be good for me to do some 'stretches', but I got much more than that. I now practice power-flow vinyasa yoga (as well as exploring other types) and feel the best that I have ever felt in my whole life. Practicing yoga has amazing benefits, both physically and mentally, but the most important thing is that I absolutely love it. It does not feel like a workout and I never have to push myself to practice it, and that is why I do it almost everyday. It is just what I do now, it is a part of my lifestyle, just like eating nutrient dense food everyday, I practice yoga.

An important thing to remember if you are trying to lose weight is, you are not going to do it just by exercising. If you do not eat properly, no matter how hard you exercise, you will not lose weight. In fact you do not even need to exercise to lose weight. Yes sure, you will get results faster and build a stronger body but if you are filling your body with traditional foods in the right portions to suit your needs, this alone will allow you to lose fat. In saying that, the health benefits of exercise make it important to include into your life, but you need to make the shift from exercising to lose weight to exercising because you enjoy it, this along with eating well, will have you see the results you are after.

Rest And Recovery

As much as exercise is great for building fitness, sculpting your body and giving you an energy boost, rest is also important. Be sure to allocate one or two days each week where you can let your body rest. The following is a list of benefits your will get from resting;

- Prevent overuse injuries
- Restore glycogen, the energy in your muscles
- Allow for muscle fibre repairs- when you exercise, particularly lifting weights and doing plyometrics, your muscles go through tiny tears. Resting will help these tears to heal and thus prevent injury and allow for greater muscle strengthening next time you exercise
- Improve fitness- allowing time for your body to rest will actually allow you to perform better the next time you exercise which means that your overall fitness can improve
- Prevent mental fatigue- your mind needs to rest as well as your body

What to do on rest days:

This is up to you. You can choose to do absolutely nothing, kick your feet up and relax.

Otherwise you can 'lightly' move you body. For example, go for a short stroll or take a yin yoga class, this is a style that just involves stretches which will also help to aid recovery in your muscles, joints and ligaments and it makes you feel amazing! It is up to you what you choose to do on your rest days, but make sure that you do allow your body to rest and recover so that it can do any healing that needs to be done and become stronger.

Other ways to rejuvenate:

Along with taking breaks from exercise, there are other ways that you can help your body repair that will help to prevent injury, allow you to exercise more effectively and make you feel fantastic.

Massage- remedial massage will help to realign muscle fibres which will release tension in the muscles, ligaments and tendons.

Chiropractic- we put a lot of pressure on our spine from our day-to-day activities and this causes it to become out of alignment which can lead to pain and discomfort. Getting adjusted will enable proper alignment of your spine, which can affect your whole body, even your immune system.

A day at the spa- we all love these. It is important to treat yourself to a facial, pedicure or body scrub/rub. You need to take care of you mind as well as your physical body.

A LOOK INTO MY PANTRY

You may be curious to know what exactly you would find in the pantry of a traditional holistic Nutritionist, so I thought I would share what you what you will find in mine.

What You Will Find in My Fridge

- Raw organic milk, cream, cheese and yoghurt from grass-fed cows. Sometimes I cannot find raw cheese and opt for pasteurised.
- Organic unsalted butter from grass-fed cows. I add my own himalayan pink salt to get all of the micronutrients and leave a small amount in the pantry so that it is easy to spread.
- Organic homemade kombucha
- Full fat organic quark from grass-fed cows. This is a creamy cheese which tastes like a mix between cottage cheese and sour cream, it is great for both sweet and savoury dishes, mashed avocado and quark is delicious.
- Organic activated nuts. In the warm months, these are best kept in the fridge to keep them fresh.
- Organic vegetables, whatever is in season
- Organic B grade maple syrup, a bottle lasts a long time in my house as it is only consumed infrequently

- Organic tahini paste
- Cold pressed Cod liver oil
- Organic eggs from pastured hens.
- Organic blanched almond meal.
- Organic berries
- Fresh fish or meat if we are having it that night
- Freshly baked bread (made with almond meal), sometimes I will leave this out on the counter, in the cooler months
- Homemade chai tea. I make a big batch every five days or so and use a milk frother to heat up a cup.

What You Will Find in My Freezer

- Organic pastured meat- beef, lamb, chicken and pork. I buy my meat in bulk from our local farmers and freeze it.
- Any meals that I have made in bulk
- Organic berries, if not in season
- Homemade bone broth

What You Will Find in My Pantry

- Organic seasonal root vegetables
- Organic seasonal fruit
- Organic onions
- Organic garlic
- Organic raw cacao powder

- Organic coconut flour
- Organic coconut (desiccated and toasted flakes)
- Expeller pressed organic virgin coconut oil
- Organic raw honey, used infrequently
- Organic brown rice syrup, also used in small amounts
- Organic nut butters
- Organic Spices
- Himalayan salt
- Organic peppercorns
- Organic coffee (for my husband, I love the aroma but I have never taken a liking to drinking it)
- Organic baking powder and baking soda
- Organic dark chocolate- a favourite is Vivani 92%. I am always trying new brands and often have an array of chocolate ranging from 75% and up to 100% cacao
- Organic tea- rooibos, many varieties of chai and other herbal teas
- Organic cold pressed extra virgin olive oil
- Organic walnut oil
- Homemade snacks
- Kombucha brewing

There you have a glimpse of the food found in my house. Eating one hundred percent organic did not happen immediately for me, I gradually made swaps with the food I bought until I could source the best places to find organic produce. Remember the order of preference when converting your kitchen into an organic one; animal produce, fruit and vegetables consumed with the skin, fruit and vegetables consumed without the skin, nuts and seeds, baking goods and other items.

FINAL WORDS

Nothing is more nourishing to the body than food raised or grown traditionally. Providing an environment that enables food to flourish will supply all the nutrients necessary to build a thriving body. That is; chemical-free, fertile soils, for plants to grow, lush green grass for animals to graze, wide open spaces for pigs to roam and grub filled fields for chickens to peck. A body that thrives is able to function efficiently, offering you the best possible chance to live a healthy, long and energetic life.

Eating traditionally, the way our ancestors did, is the most beneficial way to live. It really is quite simple, all you need to do is steer clear of absurd fad diets and eat 'real' food. By real food I mean food that is local organic and in its most natural state, such as, full fat dairy, grass-fed animal produce, eggs from pastured hens, fruit and vegetables that are in season, prepared ancient grains (if you choose) and fermented foods and beverages. In conjunction with this, we need to avoid seed oils, sugar and unprepared grains and soy. You no longer need to waste time and money spent on phony products that claim to 'shrink' you down by a gazillion dress sizes; we all know they do not work in the long run. You can be at peace knowing that by eating wholesome food, will not only allow you to be healthy on the inside, it will also show on the outside.

I am forever grateful to the farmers who farm using ethical and organic methods. They have an immense impact on the health of so many and I acknowledge them for sticking to what they believe, and farming the only way that should be allowed. The more we support these people, the more real food we will see on the market and the healthier we can be.

I acknowledge you for taking control of your health, it is, I believe, the most important thing in the world. Not only for you, but for those in your life who are important to you and want you to be happy and healthy. With this new knowledge, you are well and truly on your way to building a thriving body. Continue this journey you are on, take with you what serves you well and leave behind what has no benefit.

PRAISE TO THESE TRADITIONALFOODIES

Nina Planck- I am a big fan of Nina, she started the very first farmers market in England. Her writing is both informative and joyful to read. 'Real Food: What to Eat and Why' was the very first book I read on traditional eating and I relied a lot on her book 'Real Food for Mother and Baby: The Fertility Diet, Eating for Two, and Baby's First Foods.' when I was pregnant with Jasper. She has also written some cookbooks- 'The Farmers Market Cookbook' teaches you how to eat seasonally, when foods are best eaten and how to store and cook with them, I found this very handy. I am really looking forward to reading her latest book 'The Real Food Cookbook: Traditional Dishes for Modern Cooks' which comes out in June 2014.

Sally Fallon Morell and **Mary Enig**- Sally and Mary are a wealth of knowledge. I thoroughly enjoyed their book 'Nourishing Traditions: The Cookbook that Challenges Politically Correct Nutrition and the Diet Dictocrats' As well as 'Eat Fat, Lose Fat: The Healthy Alternative to Trans Fats', this book shows that saturated fats are essential to weight loss and health, it includes decades of research to back up their thesis. The book has a meal guide and is a great read for those looking to lose weight or improve overall health in general.

Weston A. Price Foundation- founded by Sally Fallon and Mary Enig, this non-profit organisation is dedicated to reintroducing nutrient-dense foods to the diet through education, research and activism. It has great articles including research,studies and opinion. Weston Price was a dentist who, in the 1920's and 1930s studied the dental health and development of pre-industrial populations. His findings show the detrimental impact industrialised food has had on our health, as well as how the body thrives on a traditional diet. His book 'Nutrition and Physical Degeneration' includes all of his findings.

Sarah Wilson- Sarah's autoimmune disease had her eliminate sugar from her diet forever, and she never felt better. Her story is inspiring and she is impacting the health of many. Sarah writes an enjoyable blog on her website I Quit Sugar and includes wonderful recipes. Sarah's book takes you on a step by step program on how you can quit sugar, and stay off it for life.

Pete Evans- a celebrity chef turned health coach and paleo ambassador, Pete is a true inspiration. His adoption of a traditional food diet is improving the health of so many and this is just wonderful to see. He shares great recipes in his latest book 'Healthy

Everyday' and stars in the television 'The Paleo Way'
which will air early in 2015. Pete is a wealth of
knowledge and a true leader for the future of nutrition.

Other great reads that I highly recommend;

'Primal Body, Primal Mind: Beyond the Paleo Diet for
Total Health and A Longer Life.' by Nora Gedgaudas
'Grain Brain' by David Perlmutter
'Wheat Belly' by William Davis
'Sweet Poison' and 'Toxic Oil' by David Gillespie
'Fat Chance: Beating the Odds Against Sugar, Processed
Food, Obesity and Disease'. by Robert Lustig
'The Untold Story of Milk: Green Pastures, Contented
Cows and Raw Dairy'. by Ron Schmid

GLOSSARY

Antioxidants are substances that combat free radicals (the reactive metabolic waste). Several antioxidant examples include vitamin C, vitamin E, lycopene, carotenoids and selenium.

Calcium is a mineral present in large amounts in dairy foods, such as milk, cheese and yoghurt. Also it can be found in canned salmon with bones, sardines, oysters, almonds, sesame seeds and tahini. Calcium is important for building strong bones and teeth. Having enough calcium during childhood and teenage years is very important in fighting against bone loss and osteoporosis in later life.

Calorie (Cal) is a term used for the amount of energy released when a food is burned for fuel in the body. The metric term for calories is kilojoule (kJ). One calorie equals 4.2 kilojoules.

Carbohydrates There are two main forms of carbohydrate: simple carbohydrates or sugars (such as glucose, fructose and lactose); and complex carbohydrates or starches (such as starchy vegetables, fruit, legumes, grains, rice, breads and cereals). Most carbohydrates are digested (broken down) into glucose, which is then absorbed into the bloodstream. As blood glucose levels rise, the pancreas releases a hormone called insulin. Insulin is required to move the glucose from the blood into the cells where it can be used as a source of energy.

Carotene is a substance found in some food, which is converted to vitamin A in the body. The richest food sources of beta carotene include orange and yellow fruit and vegetables.

Cholesterol may be one of two different types:
a) Blood cholesterol is a fatty substance produced by the body and carried by the blood.
b) Dietary cholesterol is found in animal foods (offal, fatty meats and poultry, eggs, full fat milk, full fat cheese etc.).

Dietary fibre is only found in plant foods. It is the part of plants not digested in the stomach and small intestine. A lot of the dietary fibre consumed is digested by bacteria in the large intestine. There are two different types of fibre:

a) Major sources of soluble fibre include fresh and dried fruits, vegetables, oats, legumes and psyllium husks.

b) Insoluble fibre acts as a stool softener and helps prevent constipation. It is found in breads, cereals, fruits, vegetables, legumes, seeds and nuts.

Energy is the amount of kilojoules or calories eaten or used. A high energy food is a high kilojoule or calorie food.

Folic acid (folate or vitamin B9) is found naturally in most plant foods, especially green leafy and other vegetables (such as spinach)

Grass Fed American Grassfed Association defines as: a) Animal having been from birth to harvest, fed on grass, legumes and forages and, b) Animals having not been: creep fed as calves, fed for extended periods in confinement, or finished on grains (as grain feeding destroys the nutritional benefits of grass fed beef).

Hydrogenation is a chemical process which makes liquid oils more saturated and solid. This process not only increases the amount of saturated fat in the oil, but also produces trans fats. Hydrogenated fats are commonly used by food manufacturers, such as in the production of biscuits, pastries, snack foods and convenience foods.

Iron is a mineral present in food in two main forms:
a) Haem iron is found in red meat, poultry and seafood. Haem iron is much better absorbed by the body than non-haem iron.
b) Non-haem iron is found in cereals, fruit (especially some dried fruits such as raisins and apricots), vegetables, legumes.
Absorption of the iron found in these foods can be increased by adding a vitamin C rich food to the meal, like fresh orange juice, or by adding a food rich in haem iron, such as lean beef or lean lamb.

Iron helps red blood cells to carry oxygen around the body. An insufficient intake of iron can lead to a condition called iron-deficient anaemia, with symptoms such as weakness, fatigue, light-headedness and shortness of breath.

Kilojoule (kJ) is a metric term for the amount of energy produced when a food is burned in the body (see calorie above).

Legume (or pulses) is the term that covers dried beans, peas and lentils. Examples include kidney beans, chick peas, split peas and baked beans.

Magnesium is a mineral found in whole grains, wholegrain breads, nuts and seeds, wheat bran, green leafy vegetables, potatoes, beans, avocados, bananas, milk, chicken, meat, and fish. Magnesium helps the body make protein and create energy. It also helps nerve and muscle function, steadies heart rhythm and helps keeps bones strong.

Monounsaturated fat monounsaturated fats or MUFAs are fatty acids that have one double bond in the fatty acid chain and all of the remainder of the carbon atoms in the chain are single-bonded. Sources include oils from olives, peanut oils; avocado; nuts and seeds.

Niacin (vitamin B3) is found in canned tuna, fish, chicken, rabbit, turkey, beef, pork, game meat, liver kidney, peanuts and peanut butter, wholegrain food products and yeast extract. Niacin helps the body convert food into energy. It is also important for nerve function and helps maintain healthy skin.

Omega-3 fats (or omega-3 fatty acids) can be divided into two groups:
a) EPA (Eicosapentaenoic acid) and DHA (Docosahexaenoic acid) are types of omega-3 polyunsaturated fats found predominantly in fish, particularly oily fish such as salmon, sardines, mackerel, trevally and tuna.
b) ALA (Alpha Linolenic Acid) is a different type of omega-3 polyunsaturated fat. Linseeds (flaxseeds) and walnuts are high in ALA.

117

Omega-3 fats are particularly important in heart health, as well as in the normal development of children's brains and nervous systems.

Phosphorus is a mineral commonly found in many foods, including dairy foods, meat, nuts, legumes, and oats. Phosphorus helps form strong bones and teeth and also helps the body make energy.

Phytic Acid is an acid $C_6H_{18}P_6O_{24}$ that occurs in cereal grains and that when ingested interferes with the intestinal absorption of various minerals (as calcium and magnesium)

Phytoestrogens are plant chemicals that have a similar structure to that of the human hormone oestrogen and which behave like weak oestrogens in the body. They are found in a variety of foods including soy drinks, soy yogurt, soy flour, soybeans, roasted soy nuts, lentils, tofu, tempeh, miso, textured vegetable protein (TVP), chickpeas, broad beans and linseed meal.

Polyunsaturated fat or PUFAS a class of fats having long carbon chains with many double bonds unsaturated with hydrogen atoms. Sources include margarine spreads and oils made from, sunflower safflower, soybean and corn oils; oily fish; shellfish; and nuts and seeds.

Potassium is a mineral found in a lot of foods. Good sources include leafy green vegetables, vine fruits (such as tomatoes, cucumbers, zucchini, eggplant and pumpkin), and root vegetables (such as potatoes with skins). Potassium is also moderately abundant in beans and peas, tree fruits (such as apples, oranges and bananas), milks and yogurts, and meats. Potassium helps with muscle and nervous system function. It also plays a role in helping the body maintain the balance of water in the blood and body tissues.

Protein is a major component of food. Good sources of protein include lean meat, fish, dairy products, eggs and legumes. Proteins are made up of smaller units called amino acids. There are 23 amino acids, eight of which are known as 'essential amino acids', meaning they cannot be made in the body and must be derived from food. Proteins are essential for building, maintaining and replacing body tissues. Your muscles, immune system and organs are made up mostly of protein.

Riboflavin (Vitamin B2) is found in liver, kidney, dairy products, eggs, meat, legumes, almonds, broccoli, asparagus, yeast extract and fortified breads and breakfast cereals. Riboflavin is essential for converting carbohydrates into energy, producing red blood cells and for healthy vision.

Saturated fat is fat that consists of triglycerides containing only saturated fatty acids. Saturated fatty acids have no double bonds between the individual carbon atoms of the fatty acid chain. Sources include full-fat dairy products, cream, butter lard, ghee.

Thiamin (vitamin B1) is a B vitamin found mainly in cereals such as wholemeal pasta and bread, brown rice, rolled oats, bulgur or cracked wheat, yeast extract and fortified breakfast cereals and bread. Thiamin plays an essential role in converting carbohydrates into energy and is necessary for the muscles, heart and nervous system to function properly.

Trans fats (or trans fatty acids) are a type of fat found naturally in small amounts in meat and some dairy products. However, the main sources of trans fats are found in foods made using processed (partially hydrogenated) vegetable oils, such as baked goods like commercial cakes, pastries and biscuits. Hydrogenation is used by a lot of food manufacturers to solidify liquid vegetable oils to make products such a margarines and shortenings. Trans fats behave like saturated fats in the body by increasing total and LDL ('bad') blood cholesterol levels. They also have the added negative effect on health of lowering HDL ('good') cholesterol. All of these changes increase your risk of heart disease and stroke.

Triglycerides are a type of fat carried in the blood. Too many triglycerides in the blood can increase the risk of heart disease.

Vitamin A is a fat-soluble vitamin found in milk, eggs, liver, fortified cereals, dark coloured orange or green vegetables.

Vitamin B6 is a B vitamin found in a wide range of foods including fish, lentils, beans, pork, poultry, beef, lamb, nuts, bananas, avocado and a variety of other fruit and vegetables. Vitamin B6 is important for normal nerve and brain function. It also helps the body break down proteins to make red blood cells.

Vitamin B12 is a B vitamin found mainly in animal foods, particularly liver and kidney. It is also found in rabbit, duck, pork, lamb, turkey, chicken, oysters and fish. Vitamin B12 helps make red blood cells and is also essential for nerve cell function.

Vitamin C (ascorbic acid) is a water-soluble vitamin found in fresh fruit (especially citrus fruit kiwi fruit, guava, pawpaw and strawberries) and vegetables (especially capsicum, Brussels sprouts, broccoli and cauliflower). Vitamin C is an antioxidant (see above), which means that it helps protect the body's cells from damage by free radicals. Vitamin C has a number of other functions such as helping the body absorb iron and calcium from the food we eat and heal wounds.. It is essential for healthy bones, teeth, gums, and blood vessels and is needed to help form collagen, a tissue that helps hold our cells together.

Vitamin D is a fat-soluble vitamin that is found in small amounts in egg yolks, fish oils and fortified foods such as milk. Most of the vitamin D that our body needs is manufactured by our body when we get sunlight on our skin. Vitamin D is important for strong bones and teeth, as it helps the body absorb bone-building calcium.

Vitamin E is a fat-soluble vitamin and antioxidant found in avocados as well as other fatty foods.

Zinc is a mineral found in many foods. Good sources include oysters and other seafood, meats, fish and poultry, dried beans, nuts, oats, bran, rice, wholemeal bread and fortified breakfast cereals. Zinc is important for normal growth and development, a healthy immune system and healing wounds.

ABOUT THE AUTHOR

Born in the south-east suburbs of Melbourne, Australia
Nutritionist and Master Fitness Trainer, Amanda Jayne
Harvey is passionate about living a life that she loves.
Growing up as a dedicated equestrian rider and

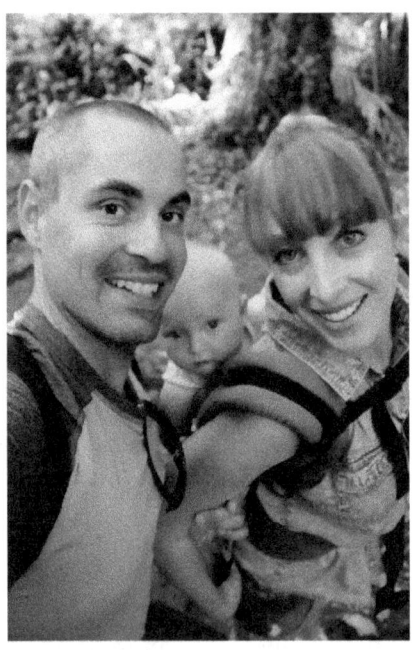

becoming a qualified veterinary nurse and equine sports
therapist, Amanda spent most of her days being active
outdoors with her horses. When she took a break to

travel the world she discovered along the way a new love for health, and a burning passion for nutrition.

Amanda is lucky enough to be married to the man of her dreams. They share the same love for travelling, hiking and yoga and welcomed the arrival of their first son, Jasper, in June 2013. Her family is her number one priority and she makes sure she spends as much time as possible with them.

Amanda keeps up to date with changes in nutritional science. She enjoys creating delicious nutrient rich recipes which, along with her blog, shares on her website "The Noble Nutritionist" and Facebook page.

Bibliography

[1] "Diet - Definition and More from the Free Merriam-Webster Dictionary." 2006. 20 Feb. 2014
<http://www.merriam-webster.com/dictionary/diet>

[2] "Types of Carbohydrates: American Diabetes Association®." 2014. 20 Feb. 2014
<http://www.diabetes.org/food-and-fitness/food/what-can-i-eat/understanding-carbohydrates/types-of-carbohydrates.html>

[3] "Living With Phytic Acid - Weston A Price Foundation." 2011. 20 Feb. 2014
<http://www.westonaprice.org/food-features/living-with-phytic-acid>

[4] "Disaccharide - Wikipedia, the free encyclopedia." 2003. 20 Feb. 2014
<http://en.wikipedia.org/wiki/Disaccharide>

[5] "Big Fat Lies: How the diet industry is making you sick, fat & poor ..." 2012. 29 Nov. 2013
<http://www.penguin.com.au/products/9780670076024/big-fat-lies-how-diet-industry-making-you-sick-fat-poor>

[6] Howard, BV. "Sugar and Cardiovascular Disease - Circulation." 2002.
<http://circ.ahajournals.org/content/106/4/523.full>

[7] Ganong, William F, and Kim E Barrett. *Review of medical physiology*. New York: McGraw-Hill Medical, 2005.

[8] Burt, Brian A, and Satishchandra Pai. "Sugar consumption and caries risk: a systematic review." *Journal of Dental Education* 65.10 (2001): 1017-1023.

126

[9] Fallon, Sally, and Mary G Enig. "Tripping lightly down the prostaglandin pathways." *Price-Pottenger Nutr. Foundation Health J* 20.3 (1996): 5-8.

[10] Vartanian, Lenny R, Marlene B Schwartz, and Kelly D Brownell. "Effects of soft drink consumption on nutrition and health: a systematic review and meta-analysis." *American Journal of Public Health* 97.4 (2007): 667-675.

[11] Bostick, Roberd M et al. "Sugar, meat, and fat intake, and non-dietary risk factors for colon cancer incidence in Iowa women (United States)." *Cancer Causes & Control* 5.1 (1994): 38-52.

[12] Gibson, S, and S Williams. "Dental Caries in Pre–School Children: Associations with Social Class, Toothbrushing Habit and Consumption of Sugars and Sugar–Containing Foods." *Caries research* 33.2 (1999): 101-113.

[13] Bellisle, F. "Functional foods and the satiety cascade." *Nutrition Bulletin* 33.1 (2008): 8-14.

[14] Bellisle, France et al. "Sweetness, satiation, and satiety." *The Journal of nutrition* 142.6 (2012): 1149S-1154S.

[15] Bornet, Francis RJ et al. "Glycaemic response to foods: impact on satiety and long-term weight regulation." *Appetite* 49.3 (2007): 535-553.

[16] "Fat | Define Fat at Dictionary.com." 2006. 21 Feb. 2014 <http://dictionary.reference.com/browse/fat>

[17] "Big Fat Lies: The Truth About Your Weight and Your Health: Glenn A ..." 2006. 21 Feb. 2014 <http://www.amazon.com/Big-Fat-Lies-Weight-Health/dp/0936077425>

[18] Borel, Patrick. "Factors affecting intestinal absorption of highly lipophilic food microconstituents (fat-soluble vitamins, carotenoids and phytosterols)." *Clinical Chemistry and Laboratory Medicine* 41.8 (2003): 979-994.

[19] Daley, CA. "A review of fatty acid profiles and antioxidant content in grass-fed ..." 2010. <http://www.ncbi.nlm.nih.gov/pubmed/20219103>

[20] Hu, Frank B, JoAnn E Manson, and Walter C Willett. "Types of dietary fat and risk of coronary heart disease: a critical review." *Journal of the American College of Nutrition* 20.1 (2001): 5-19.

[21] Risérus, Ulf, Walter C Willett, and Frank B Hu. "Dietary fats and prevention of type 2 diabetes." *Progress in lipid research* 48.1 (2009): 44-51.

[22] Lissner, Lauren, and Berit L Heitmann. "Dietary fat and obesity: evidence from epidemiology." *European journal of clinical nutrition* 49.2 (1995): 79.

[23] Mozaffarian, Dariush, Renata Micha, and Sarah Wallace. "Effects on coronary heart disease of increasing polyunsaturated fat in place of saturated fat: a systematic review and meta-analysis of randomized controlled trials." *PLoS medicine* 7.3 (2010): e1000252

[24] Hu, Frank B et al. "Dietary fat intake and the risk of coronary heart disease in women." *New England*

Bibliography

Journal of Medicine 337.21 (1997): 1491-1499.

[25] Salmeron, Jorge et al. "Dietary fat intake and risk of type 2 diabetes in women." *The American journal of clinical nutrition* 73.6 (2001): 1019-1026.

[26] Simopoulos, Artemis P, and Leslie G Cleland. *Omega-6, Omega-3 Essential Fatty Acid Ratio: The Scientific Evidence; 37 Tables.* Artemis P Simopoulos & Leslie G Cleland. Karger Publishers, 2003.

[27] Olcott, HS, and HA Mattill. "Constituents of Fats and Oils Affecting the Development of Rancidity." *Chemical Reviews* 29.2 (1941): 257-268.

[28] Erasmus, Udo. *Fats That Heal, Fats That Kill: The Complete Guide to Fats, Oils, Cholesterol and Human Health.* Book Publishing Company, 1993.

[29] "Reactive oxygen species - Wikipedia, the free encyclopedia." 2004. 21 Feb. 2014 <http://en.wikipedia.org/wiki/Reactive_oxygen_species>

[30] "Put down that doughnut: FDA takes on trans fats - CNN.com." 2013. 29 Nov. 2013

[31] Astrup, Arne et al. "The role of reducing intakes of saturated fat in the prevention of cardiovascular disease: where does the evidence stand in 2010?." *The American journal of clinical nutrition* 93.4 (2011): 684-688.

[32] Siri-Tarino, Patty W et al. "Saturated fat, carbohydrate, and cardiovascular disease." *The American journal of clinical nutrition* 91.3 (2010): 502-

509.

[33] Fallon, Sally. "Nourishing traditions: the cookbook that challenges politically correct nutrition and the diet dictocrats." (1999).

[34] Burr, George O, and Mildred M Burr. "On the nature and role of the fatty acids essential in nutrition." *Journal of Biological Chemistry* 86.2 (1930): 587-621.

[35] McCluskey, Jill J et al. "US Grass-Fed Beef: Marketing Health Benefits." *Journal of Food Distribution Research* 36.3 (2005).

[36] Pastures, Greener. "How grass-fed beef and milk contribute to healthy eating." *Cambridge, MA: Union of Concerned Scientists* (2006).

[37] Melton, SL et al. "Flavor and chemical characteristics of ground beef from grass-, forage-grain-and grain-finished steers." *Journal of Animal Science* 55.1 (1982): 77-87.

[38] Daley, Cynthia A et al. "A review of fatty acid profiles and antioxidant content in grass-fed and grain-fed beef." *Nutrition Journal* 9.1 (2010): 10.

[39] Hebeisen, Dorothea F et al. "Increased concentrations of omega-3 fatty acids in milk and platelet rich plasma of grass-fed cows." *International journal for vitamin and nutrition research. Internationale Zeitschrift fur Vitamin-und Ernahrungsforschung. Journal international de vitaminologie et de nutrition* 63.3 (1992): 229-233.

Bibliography

[40] Blake, Gavin J, and Paul M Ridker. "Novel clinical markers of vascular wall inflammation." *Circulation research* 89.9 (2001): 763-771.

[41] Jones, PJ, and Dale A Schoeller. "Evidence for diurnal periodicity in human cholesterol synthesis." *Journal of lipid research* 31.4 (1990): 667-673.

[42] "Guidelines for a Low Cholesterol, Low Saturated Fat Diet | Patient ..." 2010. 22 Feb. 2014 <http://www.ucsfhealth.org/education/guidelines_for_a_low_cholesterol_low_saturated_fat_diet/>

[43] "Cholesterol: Friend Or Foe? - Weston A Price Foundation." 2010. 22 Feb. 2014 <http://www.westonaprice.org/know-your-fats/cholesterol-friend-or-foe>

[44] Devlin, Thomas M. *Textbook of biochemistry: with clinical correlations*. Thomas M Devlin. Hoboken, NJ: John Wiley & Sons, 2011.

[45] "Metabolism - Definition and More from the Free Merriam-Webster ..." 2005. 22 Feb. 2014 <http://www.merriam-webster.com/dictionary/metabolism>

[46] Harrington, Monica. "Dangers of BPA exposure confirmed in rhesus macaques." *Lab animal* 41.11 (2012): 302.

[47] Murphy, M. "Chemicals industry is hiding dangers of BPA." *CHEMISTRY & INDUSTRY* 3 (2005): 7-7.
[48] "Calorie - Definition and More from the Free Merriam-Webster ..." 2006. 22 Feb. 2014 <http://www.merriam-

Bibliography

webster.com/dictionary/calorie>

[49] Dansinger, Michael L et al. "Comparison of the Atkins, Ornish, Weight Watchers, and Zone diets for weight loss and heart disease risk reduction: a randomized trial." *Jama* 293.1 (2005): 43-53.

[50] Hunter, David J et al. "Plasma organochlorine levels and the risk of breast cancer." *New England Journal of Medicine* 337.18 (1997): 1253-1258.

[51] Koutros, Stella et al. "Heterocyclic aromatic amine pesticide use and human cancer risk: results from the US Agricultural Health Study." *International Journal of Cancer* 124.5 (2009): 1206-1212.

[52] Hou, Lifang et al. "Environmental chemical exposures and human epigenetics." *International journal of epidemiology* 41.1 (2012): 79-105.

[53] "The Whole Soy Story: The Dark Side of America's Favorite Health ..." 2012. 22 Feb. 2014 <http://www.amazon.com/The-Whole-Soy-Story-Americas/dp/0967089751>

[54] "Big Fat Lies: The Truth About Your Weight and Your Health: Glenn A ..." 2006. 22 Feb. 2014 <http://www.amazon.com/Big-Fat-Lies-Weight-Health/dp/0936077425>

[55] "Deep Nutrition | drcate.com." 2009. 22 Feb. 2014 <http://drcate.com/deep-nutrition-the-ancient-science-of-human-engineering/>

[56] Horrocks, Lloyd A, and Young K Yeo. "Health benefits of docosahexaenoic acid (DHA)."

Pharmacological Research 40.3 (1999): 211-225.

[57] Enig, Mary G. "Health and nutritional benefits from coconut oil." *Price-Pottenger Nutr. Foundation Health J* 20.1 (1998): 1-6.

[58] Enig, Mary G. "Health and nutritional benefits from coconut oil: an important functional food for the 21st century." *AVOC Lauric Oils Symposium, Ho Chi Min City, Vietnam* 25 Apr. 1996.

[59] Banzon, Julian A, and Jose R Velasco. "Coconut: production and utilization." *Coconut: production and utilization* (1982).

[60] "Nutrition and Physical Degeneration: Weston A. Price ... - Amazon.com." 2008. 22 Feb. 2014 <http://www.amazon.com/Nutrition-Physical-Degeneration-Weston-Price/dp/0916764206>

[61] Agero, AL, and Vermén M Verallo-Rowell. "A randomized double-blind controlled trial comparing extra virgin coconut oil with mineral oil as a moisturizer for mild to moderate xerosis." *Dermatitis: contact, atopic, occupational, drug* 15.3 (2004): 109-116
.

[62] Sircar, S, and U Kansra. "Choice of cooking oils--myths and realities." *Journal of the Indian Medical Association* 96.10 (1998): 304-307.

[63] "Ferment - Definition and More from the Free Merriam-Webster ..." 2005. 22 Feb. 2014 <http://www.merriam-webster.com/dictionary/ferment>